The AuDHD Woman's Guide to Hormones and Life Transitions

Understanding Your Neurodivergent Mind Through Every Stage

Constantino Maria Porter

ISBN: 978-1-7642235-6-0

Isohan Publishing

Table of Contents

Chapter 1: The Hidden Women

Why AuDHD Is Different for Us

The waiting room buzzed with the usual sounds of clinical practice—hushed conversations, rustling papers, children fidgeting in plastic chairs. But for Sarah, the 34-year-old marketing director sitting quietly in the corner, this ordinary Tuesday represented the end of a decades-long mystery. After years of struggling with what doctors had labeled anxiety, depression, and "stress-related issues," she was finally here for an AuDHD evaluation. The path to this moment hadn't been straightforward—it never is for women like Sarah.

The story of AuDHD in women begins with a fundamental truth: we've been hiding in plain sight for generations. The term AuDHD, coined by the neurodivergent community, describes the co-occurrence of autism and ADHD—a combination found in 50-70% of autistic individuals. Yet despite affecting millions of women, this dual diagnosis remains one of the most misunderstood and underdiagnosed conditions in modern medicine.

The Masking Phenomenon and Its Metabolic Cost

The first key to understanding AuDHD in women lies in recognizing what researchers call "masking" or "camouflaging." This isn't the casual social adjustment we all make—putting on professional demeanor at work or being extra polite at dinner parties. For AuDHD women, masking represents a full-time performance that can span decades.

Case Example: Maria's Exhausting Performance

Maria, a 41-year-old teacher, described her masking experience: "Every morning, I put on what I call my 'human costume.' I practice facial expressions in the bathroom mirror. I rehearse small talk topics. I force myself to make eye contact even though it feels like staring into bright lights. By the time I get to work, I'm already running on fumes, but the day hasn't even begun."

Maria's description captures the essence of masking—the conscious and unconscious suppression of natural AuDHD traits to appear neurotypical. Research from the Frontiers in Psychiatry journal reveals that masking is significantly more common in women, with several contributing factors:

The Social Training of Girls

From early childhood, girls receive different messages about acceptable behavior. While boys might be told "boys will be boys" when they display hyperactive or disruptive behaviors, girls learn they must be socially adept, compliant, and emotionally regulated. This creates what researchers term "gendered socialization pressure"—the expectation that women should naturally excel at social communication and emotional management.

AuDHD girls quickly learn that their natural responses—stimming, direct communication, intense interests, sensory sensitivities—mark them as "different" in ways that attract negative attention. The solution? They develop sophisticated masking strategies:

- **Mimicking neurotypical behaviors**: Watching and copying how other girls interact, speak, and move
- **Rehearsing social scripts**: Preparing conversation topics and responses in advance
- **Suppressing natural responses**: Hiding stimming behaviors, forcing eye contact, containing excitement about interests
- **People-pleasing behaviors**: Becoming hyper-attuned to others' emotions and needs

The Metabolic Cost of Constant Performance

But masking comes with a severe price. The Sachscenter research describes it perfectly: imagine starting every day with your mental battery already at 50%. That's the reality for many AuDHD women. The constant effort of masking autistic traits while managing ADHD symptoms creates what researchers call "chronic energy deficit."

The metabolic cost manifests in several ways:

2

Physical Exhaustion: The body remains in a heightened state of vigilance, constantly monitoring and adjusting behavior. This chronic stress response depletes physical energy reserves.

Cognitive Overload: Mental resources that should be available for learning, creativity, and problem-solving get redirected toward maintaining the mask. Executive function suffers as cognitive bandwidth gets consumed by social performance.

Emotional Depletion: The suppression of authentic emotional responses creates internal tension. Many women describe feeling like they're constantly "performing happiness" while struggling internally.

Social Hangover: After social interactions, many AuDHD women experience what researchers term "social hangover"—a period of complete mental and physical depletion that can last hours or days.

Case Example: The Boom-and-Bust Cycle

Jennifer, a 38-year-old software developer, exemplified the typical AuDHD woman's experience: "I can hyperfocus for 12 hours straight on a coding project, completely forgetting to eat or drink. I feel like a superhero during these periods—nothing can stop me. But then I crash completely. I'll spend the next three days barely able to get dressed, let alone work. My husband calls it my 'hibernation mode.'"

Jennifer's experience illustrates the "boom-and-bust" cycle common in AuDHD women. The ADHD trait of hyperfocus provides intense productivity bursts, but the autistic need for structure and energy management gets steamrolled during these periods, leading inevitably to burnout.

How Diagnostic Criteria Miss Women's Presentations

The second major factor in AuDHD being missed in women relates to fundamental biases in diagnostic criteria. Both autism and ADHD diagnostic tools were developed primarily based on studies of boys and men, creating what researchers term "male-centric diagnostic bias."

The Numbers Tell the Story

Research from PMC reveals staggering statistics about gender bias in foundational ADHD research. Of 243 empirical studies published during a crucial period of diagnostic development, 81% of participants were male, with only 19% female. Even more striking: of 70 single-sex studies, 99.6% focused exclusively on male children.

This male-dominated research created diagnostic criteria that emphasize externalized, disruptive behaviors—the kind typically displayed by boys—while minimizing the internalized struggles more common in girls.

How ADHD Looks Different in Women

Traditional ADHD presentations focus on hyperactivity and disruptive behavior. But women with ADHD more commonly present with:

Inattentive Symptoms: Racing thoughts, difficulty focusing, mental restlessness that doesn't manifest as physical hyperactivity

Internalized Hyperactivity: Feeling like they have a "motor running inside" rather than bouncing off walls

Executive Function Struggles: Difficulty with organization, time management, and task completion that gets attributed to "laziness" or lack of motivation

Emotional Dysregulation: Intense emotional responses that get labeled as "being too sensitive" or "overreacting"

Case Example: The "Daydreamer" vs. The "Disruptor"

Consider two 8-year-olds: Jake frequently interrupts class, can't sit still, and gets in trouble for talking out of turn. Emma sits quietly, stares out the window, and seems to be daydreaming but is actually struggling to process the teacher's rapid-fire instructions while simultaneously managing sensory overload from fluorescent lights and classroom noise.

Jake gets referred for ADHD evaluation. Emma gets labeled a "daydreamer" and told to "pay better attention."

How Autism Looks Different in Women

The autism diagnostic bias is equally problematic. Women with autism often present with:

Social Motivation Despite Difficulties: Unlike the stereotypical "loner" image, many autistic women desperately want social connection but struggle with execution

Camouflaged Special Interests: Intense interests in socially acceptable topics (horses, celebrities, books) that don't trigger diagnostic attention

Internalized Repetitive Behaviors: Stimming that looks like "fidgeting" or gets disguised as socially acceptable actions

Better Surface-Level Social Skills: Learned behaviors that mask underlying social communication differences

The Autism-ADHD Intersection in Female Brains

The third crucial element involves understanding how autism and ADHD interact differently in female brains. Research published in the Journal of Attention Disorders suggests that the combination creates unique presentations that don't fit neatly into either diagnostic category.

Competing Neurological Drives

AuDHD creates a fascinating neurological paradox. The autistic brain craves predictability, routine, and structure, while the ADHD brain seeks novelty, stimulation, and change. In women, this often manifests as:

Internal Warfare: Constant tension between needing routine (autism) and craving stimulation (ADHD)

Compensatory Behaviors: Using one condition to manage the other—hyperfocus to manage sensory overload, or rigid routines to manage ADHD chaos

Masking Complexity: Needing to hide both conditions simultaneously, creating layered masking strategies

Case Example: The Routine-Seeking Procrastinator

Lisa, a 45-year-old accountant, described her daily struggle: "I need my morning routine to function—same coffee mug, same breakfast, same route to work. But I also procrastinate on important projects until the deadline pressure gives me the adrenaline rush I need to focus. I'm simultaneously the most organized and most chaotic person I know."

The Hormonal Connection

Research from Multiple sources reveals that female hormones significantly impact both autism and ADHD symptoms. Estrogen affects dopamine production and uptake—crucial for ADHD management—while also influencing sensory processing and social cognition areas affected by autism.

This creates monthly symptom fluctuations that can confuse both women and their healthcare providers. Symptoms may seem manageable during high-estrogen phases but become overwhelming during low-estrogen periods.

Reframing Traits as Neurological Differences, Not Flaws

The final piece of understanding AuDHD in women involves a fundamental shift in perspective. Instead of viewing AuDHD traits as deficits or disorders, we must recognize them as neurological differences with both challenges and strengths.

Moving Beyond the Medical Model

Traditional medical approaches focus on symptoms, deficits, and dysfunction. But the neurodiversity movement offers a different framework—one that recognizes AuDHD as a natural variation in human neurology, not a collection of problems to fix.

This doesn't mean ignoring genuine struggles or difficulties. Instead, it means understanding that many challenges stem from living in a world designed for neurotypical brains, not from inherent flaws in AuDHD brains.

The Strength-Based Approach

AuDHD women often possess remarkable abilities:

Hyperfocus and Deep Expertise: The ability to become deeply knowledgeable about areas of interest

Pattern Recognition: Enhanced ability to see connections others miss

Authentic Communication: Direct, honest communication style once masking is reduced

Creative Problem-Solving: Novel approaches to challenges

Intense Empathy: Deep emotional understanding and compassion for others

Attention to Detail: Ability to notice nuances others overlook

Environmental Awareness: Heightened sensitivity to surroundings and changes

Case Example: From Deficit to Difference

Rachel, a 37-year-old veterinarian, transformed her understanding of herself: "I used to think I was broken—too sensitive, too intense, too much work for other people. But once I understood I was AuDHD, everything shifted. My sensitivity helps me notice subtle changes in animals that other vets miss. My intense focus allows me to perform complex surgeries others find challenging. I'm not broken—I'm just different."

The Identity Integration Process

For many women, receiving an AuDHD diagnosis involves a complex process of identity integration. This includes:

Grief for the Neurotypical Self: Mourning the person they thought they were supposed to be

Relief and Validation: Finally having explanations for lifelong struggles

Reframing Past Experiences: Understanding previous challenges through a new lens

Identity Reconstruction: Building a new sense of self that incorporates AuDHD identity

Future Planning: Designing life strategies that work with, not against, their neurology

The journey toward understanding AuDHD in women requires recognition that we've been here all along—working twice as hard to appear half as capable, burning ourselves out in the pursuit of neurotypical performance standards that were never designed for our brains. The hidden women are becoming visible, and with that visibility comes the opportunity for authentic living, proper support, and the recognition that different doesn't mean deficient.

Key Insights Moving Forward

- AuDHD affects millions of women who remain undiagnosed due to masking, diagnostic bias, and misunderstanding of female presentations
- Masking carries severe metabolic costs that contribute to chronic exhaustion and burnout
- Diagnostic criteria based on male presentations systematically miss women's experiences
- The autism-ADHD intersection creates unique challenges and strengths in women
- Reframing AuDHD as neurological difference rather than deficit opens possibilities for authentic living and proper support

Understanding these foundational concepts sets the stage for exploring the complex relationship between AuDHD and hormonal fluctuations—a connection that profoundly impacts women's experiences across their lifespan.

Chapter 2: Hormones 101 for the Neurodivergent Woman

The phone call came at 2 PM on a Tuesday—precisely when Amanda had predicted it would. For the past six months, the 43-year-old graphic designer had been tracking her moods, energy levels, and ADHD symptoms with the precision of a scientist. What she discovered shocked her: her ability to focus, regulate emotions, and manage sensory input followed a predictable 28-day pattern that aligned perfectly with her menstrual cycle.

"Week one after my period, I'm a productivity machine," Amanda explained to her therapist. "Week two, I feel almost neurotypical—social situations don't drain me, I can handle the grocery store without headphones, and my ADHD medication works like it's supposed to. But week three? It's like someone flipped a switch. Suddenly I can't concentrate, every sound feels like nails on a chalkboard, and I need to script every social interaction. Week four is just survival mode."

Amanda's experience illustrates a crucial but often overlooked aspect of AuDHD in women: the profound impact of hormonal fluctuations on neurological functioning. Understanding this relationship isn't just academic—it's essential for managing symptoms, planning treatments, and designing life strategies that work with, rather than against, your body's natural rhythms.

Estrogen's Effect on Dopamine and Sensory Processing

The relationship between hormones and neurodivergence begins with understanding how estrogen—the primary female sex hormone—directly influences brain chemistry and functioning. Research from the Reproductive Health Research Institute reveals that estrogen has profound effects on neurotransmitter systems, particularly dopamine, which plays a central role in both ADHD and autism.

The Estrogen-Dopamine Connection

Estrogen's impact on dopamine is multifaceted and powerful. According to research published in Multiple scientific journals, estrogen:

- **Increases dopamine synthesis**: More dopamine gets produced when estrogen levels are higher
- **Decreases dopamine degradation**: Dopamine stays active longer in the presence of estrogen
- **Reduces dopamine reuptake**: Less dopamine gets reabsorbed, leaving more available for use
- **Stimulates dopamine receptor production**: More receptors mean better dopamine utilization

For AuDHD women, this relationship is particularly significant. ADHD involves difficulties with dopamine processing—not necessarily low dopamine, but problems with how the brain uses available dopamine. When estrogen levels are high, these processing difficulties improve. When estrogen drops, ADHD symptoms worsen.

Case Example: The Cyclical ADHD Experience

Consider Maria's monthly experience. During days 7-14 of her cycle (when estrogen peaks before ovulation), her Adderall prescription works exactly as intended. She can focus for hours, manage multiple tasks efficiently, and feels mentally sharp. But during days 21-28 (when estrogen plummets before menstruation), the same medication dose feels ineffective. She describes it as "taking a sugar pill instead of stimulant medication."

This isn't imaginary or psychological—it's neurochemical. Lower estrogen means less effective dopamine transmission, making ADHD medications less efficient and symptoms more prominent.

Estrogen and Sensory Processing

The estrogen-brain connection extends beyond dopamine to sensory processing systems—a crucial consideration for autistic women. Research from the ADDitude Magazine and menopause specialists reveals that estrogen influences:

11

Sensory Threshold Regulation: Higher estrogen levels correlate with better sensory filtering and integration

Neuroplasticity: Estrogen supports brain adaptation and learning, helping develop coping strategies

Stress Response: Estrogen modulates the hypothalamic-pituitary-adrenal axis, affecting stress reactivity

Sleep Architecture: Estrogen influences sleep quality, which directly impacts sensory processing capacity

During high-estrogen phases, many AuDHD women report improved sensory tolerance. Sounds seem less overwhelming, lights feel less harsh, and clothing textures become more manageable. Conversely, during low-estrogen phases, sensory sensitivities can become debilitating.

Case Example: The Grocery Store Test

Jenny, a 35-year-old programmer, uses grocery shopping as her personal hormone barometer: "During the first half of my cycle, I can handle Target on a Saturday afternoon—music, chatter, fluorescent lights, all of it. I might even enjoy it. But the week before my period? I need noise-canceling headphones, sunglasses, and a detailed list just to survive a quick trip to the corner store. It's like someone turned up the volume on the entire world."

Monthly Symptom Fluctuations and Pattern Tracking

Understanding monthly hormonal patterns requires knowledge of the menstrual cycle's four distinct phases, each characterized by different hormone levels and corresponding neurological effects.

Phase 1: Menstrual Phase (Days 1-5)

During menstruation, both estrogen and progesterone are at their lowest levels. For AuDHD women, this often represents the most challenging time:

ADHD Symptoms: Poor concentration, increased impulsivity, time management difficulties, emotional dysregulation

Autism Symptoms: Heightened sensory sensitivities, increased need for routine, social exhaustion, stimming behaviors more prominent

Physical Effects: Fatigue, pain sensitivity, sleep disruption

Cognitive Effects: "Brain fog," memory difficulties, reduced executive function

Case Example: The Menstrual Shutdown

Sarah, a 29-year-old teacher, describes her menstrual phase experience: "I call it my monthly shutdown. I can barely handle normal conversation, let alone manage a classroom of 25 kids. The fluorescent lights feel like torture, every sound is amplified, and I lose the ability to switch between tasks. I've learned to plan my easiest lessons during this time and avoid social commitments entirely."

Phase 2: Follicular Phase (Days 6-13)

As estrogen begins rising after menstruation, many AuDHD women experience gradual improvement in symptoms:

ADHD Improvements: Better focus, improved medication effectiveness, increased motivation, better emotional regulation

Autism Benefits: Reduced sensory sensitivities, improved social stamina, more flexible thinking

Energy Changes: Gradual increase in physical and mental energy

Mood Stabilization: Reduced anxiety and depression, improved emotional resilience

Phase 3: Ovulatory Phase (Days 14-16)

Peak estrogen levels often correlate with optimal functioning for AuDHD women:

Cognitive Peak: Best focus, memory, and executive function

Sensory Comfort: Highest sensory tolerance levels

Social Ease: Most comfortable with social interactions and changes in routine

Medication Efficiency: Stimulant medications work most effectively

Phase 4: Luteal Phase (Days 17-28)

As estrogen drops and progesterone rises, then both hormones plummet, symptoms typically worsen:

ADHD Resurgence: Return of concentration difficulties, impulsivity, emotional dysregulation

Autism Intensification: Increased sensory sensitivities, greater need for routine, social exhaustion

Premenstrual Dysphoric Disorder (PMDD): 45% of AuDHD women experience PMDD compared to 28% of neurotypical women

Physical Symptoms: Increased pain sensitivity, sleep disruption, fatigue

The Progesterone Effect

Progesterone's role in AuDHD symptoms is complex and often counterintuitive. While estrogen generally improves neurological functioning, progesterone can have opposing effects:

GABA Activation: Progesterone increases GABA (the brain's "brake pedal"), which can feel calming but may also:

- Reduce the positive effects of estrogen
- Make stimulant medications less effective
- Increase mental fatigue and "brain fog"
- Worsen inattention symptoms

Why AuDHD "Worsens" at Hormonal Transitions

The perception that AuDHD symptoms worsen at certain life stages isn't imaginary—it's based on real neurochemical changes that occur during major hormonal transitions. Understanding these transitions helps explain why many women receive their first AuDHD diagnosis during perimenopause or after major life events.

Puberty: The First Challenge

Adolescence marks the beginning of hormonal fluctuations that can unmask previously manageable AuDHD symptoms. Research shows that girls often experience symptom onset or worsening during puberty due to:

Organizational Effects: Hormones permanently alter brain structure during development

Activational Effects: Monthly hormone cycles begin affecting daily functioning

Increased Demands: Academic and social expectations increase just as neurological stability decreases

Case Example: The Straight-A Student's Decline

Rebecca was a stellar elementary student—organized, compliant, and academically successful. But seventh grade brought chaos: "Suddenly I couldn't keep track of assignments across six different classes. My locker was a disaster. I'd forget to turn in completed homework. My parents thought I was just being lazy or rebellious, but I felt like I was drowning."

What Rebecca and her parents didn't understand was that puberty had introduced hormonal variability that overwhelmed her compensatory systems. The rigid elementary school structure had masked her executive function difficulties, but middle school's complexity exposed them.

Pregnancy and Postpartum: Extreme Fluctuations

Pregnancy represents the most dramatic hormonal changes a woman's body can experience, with corresponding effects on AuDHD symptoms:

First Trimester: Rapid hormone increases can worsen nausea sensitivity and emotional regulation in AuDHD women

Second Trimester: Many women experience symptom improvement as hormones stabilize at high levels

Third Trimester: Continued high hormones often maintain improved functioning

Postpartum Crash: The dramatic hormone drop after delivery can trigger severe symptom resurgence

Research from ADDitude Magazine reveals that 98% of women discontinue ADHD medications during pregnancy, often making it difficult to separate hormonal effects from medication withdrawal effects.

Perimenopause: The Storm Before the Calm

Perimenopause—the transitional period before menopause—often represents the most challenging time for AuDHD women. Unlike the gradual decline once believed, recent research shows perimenopause involves erratic hormone fluctuations that can wreak havoc on neurological functioning.

The Estrogen Roller Coaster: Estrogen levels don't decline smoothly but instead swing wildly from very high to very low, sometimes within days

Unpredictable Symptoms: The monthly patterns women relied on for symptom management become unreliable

Medication Challenges: Previously effective medications may become ineffective during low-estrogen phases

Sleep Disruption: Hot flashes and night sweats compound existing sleep difficulties

Case Example: The Executive's Crisis

Patricia, a 48-year-old marketing executive, had managed her undiagnosed AuDHD for decades through rigid routines and overwork. Perimenopause shattered her coping systems: "I'd go into important meetings and forget key points I'd prepared. I couldn't handle the office noise that never bothered me before. Some days I felt like my old self, others like I was losing my mind. My husband suggested I was just stressed, but I knew something fundamental had changed."

Creating Personalized Hormone-Symptom Trackers

Understanding your personal hormone-symptom patterns requires systematic tracking and analysis. Effective tracking systems capture multiple variables across time to reveal meaningful patterns.

Essential Tracking Elements

A comprehensive hormone-symptom tracker should include:

Daily Ratings (1-10 scale):

- Overall energy level
- Concentration/focus ability
- Emotional regulation
- Sensory sensitivity
- Social tolerance
- Physical comfort
- Sleep quality

ADHD-Specific Symptoms:

- Attention span
- Impulsivity control
- Task completion ability
- Time management
- Medication effectiveness

Autism-Specific Symptoms:

- Sensory overload incidents
- Social exhaustion
- Need for routine/predictability
- Stimming frequency
- Special interest engagement

Physical Symptoms:

- Menstrual cycle day
- Physical pain levels
- Appetite changes
- Exercise tolerance

Environmental Factors:

- Sleep duration/quality
- Stress levels

- Major life events
- Medication changes

Digital Tracking Tools

Several apps and digital tools can facilitate hormone-symptom tracking:

Cycle Tracking Apps: Modified to include neurological symptoms alongside traditional menstrual tracking

Mood Tracking Apps: Adapted to capture ADHD and autism symptoms rather than just mood

Custom Spreadsheets: Allow complete customization but require more setup time

Wearable Devices: Can track sleep, heart rate variability, and activity levels automatically

Case Example: The Revelation Through Data

After six months of tracking, Lisa discovered her pattern: "I always thought I was just 'moody' and unpredictable. But the data showed clear patterns. My ADHD medication worked best on days 8-15 of my cycle. My sensory sensitivities peaked the week before my period. Armed with this information, I could finally make sense of my experiences and plan accordingly."

Pattern Analysis Techniques

Once you've collected several months of data, look for:

Cyclical Patterns: Symptoms that correlate with menstrual cycle phases

Medication Interactions: How hormone fluctuations affect medication effectiveness

Environmental Triggers: Factors that worsen symptoms during vulnerable phases

Protective Factors: Strategies that help during challenging phases

Seasonal Variations: How light exposure and seasonal changes interact with hormonal effects

Using Patterns for Life Planning

Pattern recognition enables strategic life planning:

Scheduling Flexibility: Plan demanding tasks during high-functioning phases

Accommodation Timing: Request accommodations during predictably difficult periods

Medication Adjustments: Work with providers to modify dosing based on cycle phases

Self-Care Intensification: Increase support during vulnerable periods

Communication Strategies: Help partners and colleagues understand pattern-based needs

The relationship between hormones and AuDHD represents one of the most significant yet underrecognized factors in women's neurological experiences. As Amanda discovered through her meticulous tracking, understanding these patterns transformed her from feeling like a victim of unpredictable symptoms to an informed advocate for her own neurological needs.

This foundational understanding of hormone-brain interactions provides the framework for navigating the specific challenges and opportunities presented at each life stage. The journey continues as we explore how these principles apply to the unique transitions women face from adolescence through menopause and beyond.

Reflections on Hormonal Awareness

The intersection of hormones and neurodivergence in women represents a frontier of understanding that has been neglected for far too long. Women like Amanda, Maria, and Patricia are not unusual— they represent millions who have struggled to understand their cyclical symptoms without proper frameworks or support.

Recognition of hormonal influences on AuDHD symptoms opens new possibilities for treatment, accommodation, and life planning. Rather than accepting unpredictable symptom fluctuations as inevitable, women can now develop informed strategies that work with their body's natural rhythms.

The journey toward hormonal awareness requires patience, systematic observation, and often, advocacy with healthcare providers who may not yet understand these connections. But the payoff—the ability to predict, prepare for, and manage neurological fluctuations— represents a fundamental shift from reactive coping to proactive thriving.

Key Insights for Neurological Navigation

- Estrogen directly influences dopamine function, making ADHD symptoms cyclical rather than constant
- Monthly hormone fluctuations create predictable patterns in both ADHD and autism symptoms
- Major hormonal transitions often unmask previously manageable AuDHD traits
- Personalized tracking reveals individual patterns that enable strategic life planning
- Understanding hormone-brain connections transforms random suffering into manageable challenges

Chapter 3: The Teen Years - Puberty Meets Neurodivergence

The text message arrived at 11:47 PM on a Tuesday—Sarah had been counting. Her 14-year-old daughter Emma had barricaded herself in her bedroom again, refusing to come out for dinner, homework, or even the family movie night they'd planned for weeks. The note slipped under the door read simply: "Everything feels too loud and too much. I can't do this anymore."

Just two years ago, Emma had been their family's organizational queen—color-coding school supplies, maintaining perfect grades, and charming teachers with her mature vocabulary and thoughtful questions. Now, she was failing three classes, crying over homework that should take 20 minutes, and experiencing daily meltdowns that left the entire family walking on eggshells.

What Sarah didn't yet understand was that her daughter was experiencing the perfect storm of AuDHD meeting adolescence—a collision that transforms previously manageable differences into overwhelming challenges that reshape both brain and body.

Hormonal Amplification of AuDHD Traits

The teenage years represent one of the most dramatic neurological upheavals in human development. For AuDHD girls, puberty doesn't just bring the typical challenges of adolescence—it fundamentally amplifies every trait, sensitivity, and struggle they've been managing since childhood.

The Hormonal Revolution

Research from ADDitude Magazine reveals that girls with ADHD typically begin puberty between ages 9 and 11, getting their first periods between ages 11 and 14. But unlike neurotypical girls, those with AuDHD experience what researchers call "symptom amplification"—their core traits become magnified in ways that can be startling to both teens and their families.

The mechanism behind this amplification lies in how hormones interact with neurotransmitter systems. As estrogen and progesterone levels begin their monthly dance, they directly affect dopamine production and uptake—the very neurotransmitter most affected in ADHD brains. Simultaneously, these hormonal fluctuations impact sensory processing, emotional regulation, and stress response systems that are already atypical in autistic brains.

Case Example: The Straight-A Student's Collapse

Meredith had been the model student through elementary school—quiet, compliant, and academically successful. She compensated for her ADHD symptoms through rigid routines and people-pleasing behaviors that masked her autistic traits. But seventh grade brought a different story.

"It was like watching our daughter disappear," her mother recalled. "One month she was organizing her binders by color and turning in every assignment early. The next month, she couldn't remember to bring home her textbooks. She'd spend three hours crying over math homework that should have taken 20 minutes."

What Meredith and her family didn't realize was that puberty had introduced hormonal variability that overwhelmed her compensatory systems. The rigid structure of elementary school had masked her executive function difficulties, but middle school's complexity—six different teachers, rotating schedules, and increased social demands—exposed traits that had been successfully hidden for years.

The hormonal changes created a cascade of effects:

Emotional Dysregulation Intensification: The already heightened emotional responses typical of AuDHD became even more extreme during hormonal fluctuations. Tasks that previously caused mild frustration now triggered complete meltdowns.

Sensory System Overhaul: Hormonal changes alter sensory processing thresholds. Sounds that were manageable became unbearable. Clothing textures that were tolerable became torturous. Lights seemed brighter, crowds felt more overwhelming.

Executive Function Breakdown: The organizational systems that worked in elementary school—when life was simpler and more predictable—couldn't adapt to the increased demands and hormonal chaos of adolescence.

Case Example: The Social Masking Crisis

Jasmine had spent years perfecting her social mask—studying other girls like a scientist, memorizing conversation scripts, and forcing herself to make eye contact even when it felt painful. But at 13, the mask began to crack under hormonal pressure.

"I felt like I was acting in a play every single day," Jasmine explained years later. "But suddenly, I couldn't remember my lines. The effort it took to appear normal was exhausting me completely. I'd come home from school and collapse for hours."

Jasmine's experience reflects a common pattern: the metabolic cost of masking becomes unsustainable during adolescence. The additional cognitive load of managing hormonal fluctuations, combined with increased social complexity, overwhelms the mental resources available for maintaining neurotypical performance.

The Boom-and-Bust Intensification

For AuDHD teens, the typical boom-and-bust cycle of hyperfocus and burnout becomes more extreme during hormonal fluctuations. Research shows that during high-estrogen phases, girls may experience enhanced focus and productivity—leading to periods where they appear to be thriving. But during low-estrogen phases, the crash becomes more severe.

Case Example: The Perfectionist's Pendulum

Aria, 15, described her monthly experience: "For about two weeks each month, I'm unstoppable. I'll hyperfocus on art projects for 8 hours straight, get ahead on all my schoolwork, and feel like I can conquer the world. Then something shifts, and I can barely brush my teeth. My executive function just disappears. Teachers think I'm lazy because they see the high-functioning version of me and don't understand why I can't maintain it."

This pattern creates particular challenges for AuDHD teens because:

1. **Performance Expectations**: Adults see the high-functioning periods and expect that level of performance consistently
2. **Internal Shame**: Teens internalize the belief that they should be able to maintain peak performance at all times
3. **Accommodation Resistance**: Because they can function well sometimes, teens and families may resist seeking accommodations or support

Academic and Social Navigation Strategies

The academic and social demands of adolescence require AuDHD teens to develop new strategies that account for their changing brains and increased environmental complexity.

Academic Flexibility Framework

Traditional academic approaches assume consistent performance capacity—but AuDHD teens need systems that accommodate their cyclical functioning patterns.

The Energy-Based Planning System

Rather than fixed schedules, AuDHD teens benefit from energy-based academic planning:

High-Energy Days: Schedule challenging tasks like new learning, complex projects, and difficult conversations during predicted high-functioning periods.

Maintenance Days: Use moderate-energy periods for review, practice, and routine tasks that don't require peak cognitive resources.

Recovery Days: Build in low-demand activities like organizational tasks, creative pursuits, or rest without guilt or pressure.

The Academic Accommodation Toolkit

Effective accommodations for AuDHD teens go beyond traditional ADHD supports:

Sensory Accommodations: Noise-canceling headphones, alternative seating options, modified lighting, and movement breaks to prevent sensory overload.

Executive Function Supports: Visual schedules, task breakdown templates, assignment trackers, and regular check-ins that account for fluctuating cognitive capacity.

Communication Accommodations: Written instructions to supplement verbal directions, extra processing time, and clear expectations that reduce uncertainty and anxiety.

Flexible Deadlines: Recognition that hormone-influenced cognitive fluctuations may require deadline adjustments during low-functioning periods.

Social Navigation Strategies

Adolescent social environments become exponentially more complex, requiring AuDHD teens to develop sophisticated navigation skills.

The Social Energy Budget

AuDHD teens need to understand and manage their social energy as a finite resource:

Social Energy Assessment: Daily check-ins to gauge available social capacity before engaging in interactions.

Selective Socializing: Choosing quality over quantity in social interactions, focusing energy on meaningful relationships rather than trying to maintain broad social networks.

Recovery Planning: Building in downtime after social events to prevent overwhelm and burnout.

The Authentic Relationship Approach

Rather than trying to maintain masks for everyone, AuDHD teens can develop tiered relationships:

Safe People: Trusted individuals with whom they can unmask and be authentic without performance pressure.

Neutral Interactions: Acquaintances who require minimal masking for brief, specific interactions.

Performance Contexts: Situations where masking is necessary and time-limited, with clear recovery plans.

Supporting AuDHD Daughters Effectively

Parents and families play crucial roles in supporting AuDHD daughters through the turbulent teenage years. Effective support requires understanding, flexibility, and advocacy skills.

Understanding the Internal Experience

Many parents struggle to understand their AuDHD daughter's experience because her challenges may not match stereotypical presentations of autism or ADHD.

Case Example: The "Drama Queen" Misunderstanding

Rachel's parents initially dismissed her emotional meltdowns as typical teenage drama. "She'd cry for hours over things that seemed minor to us," her mother admitted. "We thought she was being manipulative or attention-seeking. We had no idea she was experiencing genuine neurological overwhelm."

The shift came when Rachel's therapist explained sensory processing differences and emotional dysregulation. "Once we understood that her brain processes emotions and sensations differently, we could respond with support instead of frustration."

The Validation-First Approach

AuDHD teens need validation before solutions. Their experiences are real and challenging, even if they don't make sense to neurotypical perspectives.

Validation Language: "That sounds really overwhelming," "I can see you're struggling," "Your feelings make sense given what you're experiencing."

Avoid Minimizing: "It's not that bad," "Other kids handle this fine," "You just need to try harder" - these responses increase shame and shut down communication.

Collaborative Problem-Solving: Work with your daughter to develop solutions rather than imposing strategies that work for neurotypical teens.

Environmental Modifications

Creating supportive home environments requires attention to sensory, organizational, and emotional needs:

Sensory Sanctuary: Ensure your daughter has access to quiet, low-stimulation spaces for recovery and regulation.

Organizational Systems: Develop visual systems for tracking tasks, schedules, and responsibilities that account for executive function challenges.

Flexible Expectations: Adapt family routines and expectations to accommodate cycling energy levels and functioning capacity.

Communication Strategies: Establish clear, predictable communication patterns that reduce uncertainty and anxiety.

Educational Advocacy

Parents must become advocates for appropriate accommodations and understanding in school settings:

Documentation Development: Work with healthcare providers to document your daughter's needs and obtain formal accommodations through 504 plans or IEPs.

Educator Education: Provide teachers with information about how AuDHD presents in girls, as many educators are only familiar with male presentations.

Progress Monitoring: Regularly assess whether accommodations are effective and adjust as needed based on your daughter's changing needs.

Crisis Planning: Develop clear plans for managing meltdowns, sensory overload, and other challenges that may arise in school settings.

Building Early Resilience and Self-Advocacy

The teenage years provide crucial opportunities for AuDHD girls to develop self-awareness, self-acceptance, and advocacy skills that will serve them throughout their lives.

Identity Development and Acceptance

AuDHD teens need support in developing positive neurodivergent identity rather than seeing themselves as flawed or broken.

Strength-Based Framing: Help teens identify and celebrate their AuDHD-related strengths—intense interests, attention to detail, creativity, empathy, and unique perspectives.

Neurodiversity Education: Provide information about neurodiversity, famous neurodivergent individuals, and the value of neurological differences.

Community Connection: Connect teens with other neurodivergent young people through support groups, online communities, or advocacy organizations.

Case Example: From Shame to Strength

At 16, Zoe described her transformation: "I spent years thinking I was broken—too sensitive, too intense, too different. But learning about neurodiversity changed everything. Now I see my intense interests as superpowers. My sensitivity helps me create art that moves people. My attention to detail helps me excel in science. I'm not broken—I'm just wired differently."

Self-Advocacy Skill Development

AuDHD teens need concrete skills for advocating for their needs in various environments:

Need Identification: Help teens recognize their own patterns, triggers, and support needs through tracking and reflection exercises.

Communication Scripts: Develop templates for requesting accommodations, explaining needs, and setting boundaries.

Rights Education: Teach teens about their legal rights to accommodations in educational and employment settings.

Practice Opportunities: Role-play advocacy scenarios in safe environments before teens need to use these skills independently.

The Accommodation Request Toolkit

Effective self-advocacy requires teens to articulate their needs clearly:

Sensory Needs: "I need noise-canceling headphones during tests because auditory distractions make it impossible for me to concentrate."

Executive Function Support: "I work better with written instructions because I have difficulty processing verbal directions when I'm overwhelmed."

Social Accommodations: "I need advance notice of changes to routines because unexpected changes cause me significant anxiety."

Recovery Needs: "I need breaks between high-stimulation activities to prevent sensory overload."

Building Support Networks

AuDHD teens need diverse support networks that include family, friends, professionals, and community connections:

Professional Support: Therapists, coaches, and healthcare providers who understand neurodivergent presentations in females.

Peer Support: Other neurodivergent teens who can provide understanding, acceptance, and practical strategies.

Adult Mentors: Neurodivergent adults who can model successful self-advocacy and life management.

Family Education: Family members who understand and support their neurodivergent needs without judgment.

The teenage years for AuDHD girls represent both the greatest challenge and the greatest opportunity. While hormonal changes amplify every difficulty they've been managing, this period also provides the chance to develop authentic self-awareness, effective strategies, and strong advocacy skills.

Success during this phase isn't measured by neurotypical standards of consistent performance or social conformity. Instead, it's defined by the development of self-acceptance, effective coping strategies, and the ability to advocate for needed supports. AuDHD teens who receive understanding, appropriate accommodations, and strength-based support during adolescence are positioned to thrive as they move into young adulthood.

The key is recognizing that what looks like regression or failure may actually be the natural result of attempting to maintain unsustainable masking and compensatory strategies. When families and schools provide appropriate support and accommodations, AuDHD teens can redirect their energy from survival to growth, developing into confident, self-aware young adults who understand their needs and know how to advocate for them.

The Path Forward

Navigating adolescence with AuDHD requires a fundamental shift in expectations and approaches. Rather than trying to force teens to fit neurotypical molds, successful support involves meeting them where they are, accommodating their differences, and empowering them to develop authentic, sustainable ways of engaging with the world.

This foundation of understanding and support becomes crucial as AuDHD young women transition into the next phase of life— emerging adulthood—where they'll face new challenges around independence, relationships, and career development.

Essential Strategies for Teenage Success

- Hormonal fluctuations amplify all AuDHD traits, requiring flexible approaches to support and expectations
- Academic success requires energy-based planning and comprehensive accommodations beyond traditional ADHD supports
- Social navigation skills must account for limited social energy and the unsustainability of constant masking
- Family support needs to focus on validation, environmental modifications, and educational advocacy
- Self-advocacy development during adolescence creates the foundation for lifelong success and self-acceptance

Chapter 4: Young Adulthood - College, Career, and Relationships

The acceptance letter arrived on a Tuesday in March—thick, cream-colored paper that felt substantial in Maya's hands. She'd been accepted to her dream college with a partial scholarship, validation of years of academic excellence achieved through rigid routines and exhausting perfectionism. But as she held the letter, an unexpected wave of panic washed over her.

"Everyone else was celebrating," Maya recalled years later. "My parents were crying happy tears, my friends were congratulating me, but all I could think was: How am I going to survive without my color-coded schedule, my quiet bedroom sanctuary, and my mom's executive function backup system?"

Maya's reaction wasn't unusual. For AuDHD young women, the transition to college and career represents both tremendous opportunity and significant challenge. The very traits that helped them succeed in structured environments can become obstacles in the complex, unpredictable world of emerging adulthood.

Managing Increased Executive Function Demands

Young adulthood brings a perfect storm of executive function challenges that can overwhelm even the most accomplished AuDHD women. The transition from supported environments to independence requires managing multiple domains simultaneously—academic performance, living skills, social relationships, financial responsibility, and future planning.

The Executive Function Paradox

Many AuDHD women experience what researchers call the "executive function paradox" during emerging adulthood. They may have developed sophisticated compensatory strategies that worked in

34

childhood and adolescence, but these systems often prove inadequate for the complexity of adult responsibilities.

Case Example: The Organized Student's Chaos

Jennifer had been the most organized student in her high school—elaborate planner systems, color-coded notes, and never a missed assignment. But six weeks into college, she was failing three classes despite spending 60 hours a week studying.

"I had systems for everything in high school," Jennifer explained. "But college was different. I had to manage my own schedule across six different classes, remember to eat, do laundry, maintain relationships, work part-time, and figure out my major. My old systems couldn't handle that much complexity."

Jennifer's experience reflects the challenge many AuDHD women face: their compensation strategies were developed for simpler environments and don't scale up to adult demands.

The Perfectionism Trap

Many AuDHD women develop perfectionist tendencies as compensation for executive function challenges. This perfectionism can become counterproductive in college and career settings where "good enough" often serves better than perfect.

All-or-Nothing Thinking: AuDHD women may believe they must complete tasks perfectly or not at all, leading to procrastination and overwhelm.

Hyperfocus Exhaustion: The tendency to hyperfocus on projects can lead to burnout and neglect of other important areas.

Comparison Trap: Comparing their internal struggles to others' external appearances of effortless success increases shame and isolation.

Building Sustainable Executive Function Systems

Effective executive function management for AuDHD adults requires systems that accommodate cognitive fluctuations, energy limitations, and sensory needs.

The Energy-Based Planning System

Rather than traditional time management, AuDHD women benefit from energy-based approaches:

Daily Energy Assessment: Morning check-ins to assess cognitive capacity, emotional regulation, and sensory tolerance.

Task Matching: Pairing high-demand tasks with high-energy periods and routine tasks with low-energy times.

Buffer Time: Building in extra time for transitions, unexpected challenges, and recovery periods.

The External Brain System

AuDHD adults need robust external systems to supplement internal executive function:

Digital Tools: Apps for task management, schedule coordination, and reminder systems that account for ADHD time blindness.

Visual Systems: Calendars, charts, and organizers that make abstract concepts concrete and manageable.

Backup Systems: Multiple ways to track important information and deadlines to prevent single-point failures.

Case Example: The Digital Native's Solution

Sarah, a college junior with AuDHD, developed what she called her "digital executive assistant":

"I use five different apps that all sync together. My calendar blocks time for everything—classes, meals, homework, and recovery time. My task manager breaks big projects into tiny steps with deadlines. My habit tracker helps me maintain routines. My mood tracker helps me predict when I'll need extra support. It sounds complicated, but it's actually simpler than trying to keep everything in my head."

Dating, Disclosure, and Relationship Dynamics

Romantic relationships present unique challenges for AuDHD young women, who must navigate disclosure decisions, communication differences, and the energy demands of intimate partnerships.

The Disclosure Dilemma

AuDHD women face complex decisions about when and how to disclose their neurodivergence to romantic partners. The timing and approach can significantly impact relationship development.

Early Disclosure Challenges: Revealing neurodivergence too early may lead to premature judgments or fetishization of differences.

Late Disclosure Risks: Waiting too long can feel deceptive and may make partners feel excluded from an important aspect of identity.

Gradual Revelation Strategy: Many successful relationships involve gradual disclosure as trust and understanding develop.

Case Example: The Authenticity Journey

Emma described her dating evolution: "In my early twenties, I tried to hide everything. I'd mask completely on dates, which was exhausting and unsustainable. Then I went through a phase of leading with my diagnosis, which scared people away. Now I focus on being authentic about my needs and preferences without necessarily labeling them immediately."

Emma's approach involved:

- Being honest about sensory preferences ("I prefer quiet restaurants")
- Communicating clearly about social energy ("I need to leave by 10 PM")
- Explaining routines without apologizing ("I like to plan activities in advance")
- Gradually sharing more about her neurodivergence as relationships deepened

Communication Style Differences

AuDHD women often have communication patterns that differ from neurotypical expectations, which can create misunderstandings in romantic relationships.

Direct Communication: Autistic directness can be misinterpreted as rudeness or lack of empathy.

Processing Time: Needing time to process complex emotional conversations may be seen as disengagement.

Literal Interpretation: Taking things literally can lead to misunderstandings about implied meanings.

Emotional Regulation: Difficulty managing emotional responses may be misunderstood as volatility or instability.

Building Successful Relationship Dynamics

AuDHD women in successful relationships often develop specific strategies for managing relationship dynamics:

The User Manual Approach

Some couples find it helpful to create "user manuals" for each other:

Sensory Preferences: "I get overwhelmed in crowds, so let's agree on exit strategies for parties."

Communication Needs: "When I'm upset, I need time to process before discussing solutions."

Support Strategies: "During difficult periods, I'm most helped by practical support rather than emotional processing."

Recovery Needs: "I need alone time after social events, and it's not about you."

Case Example: The Partnership Model

Alex and Jordan developed what they called a "neurodivergent partnership model":

"We stopped trying to have a 'normal' relationship and started designing one that works for both of us," Alex explained. "Jordan understands that I need structure and predictability, so we plan dates in advance and stick to routines that work. I understand that they need spontaneity sometimes, so we build in flexibility within our structure."

Their strategies included:

- Weekly relationship check-ins to address issues before they became problems
- Clear agreements about social obligations and energy management
- Separate bedrooms to accommodate different sleep and sensory needs
- Explicit appreciation for each other's neurodivergent traits

Career Selection Honoring Neurodivergent Strengths

Career development for AuDHD women requires understanding both their unique strengths and their accommodation needs, then finding professional environments that leverage the former while supporting the latter.

Identifying AuDHD Career Strengths

AuDHD women often possess combinations of strengths that can be professionally advantageous:

Hyperfocus Ability: Capacity for deep, sustained concentration on interesting projects.

Pattern Recognition: Enhanced ability to notice details, inconsistencies, and systemic issues.

Creative Problem-Solving: Ability to approach challenges from unique angles and develop innovative solutions.

Empathy and Understanding: Deep emotional understanding that benefits helping professions.

Systematic Thinking: Ability to create and maintain organized systems and processes.

Research and Analysis Skills: Capacity for thorough investigation and detailed analysis.

Case Example: The Accidental Entrepreneur

Lisa discovered her career path through necessity rather than planning:

"I couldn't handle traditional office environments—the noise, the interruptions, the unclear expectations. I kept getting fired from jobs I was technically good at because I couldn't manage the social and sensory aspects. Finally, I started freelancing as a data analyst, working from home with clients who just wanted good work delivered on time."

Lisa's freelance business grew into a successful consulting firm because she could:

- Control her work environment to optimize focus and minimize distractions
- Structure projects around her energy patterns and hyperfocus abilities
- Work with detail-oriented tasks that matched her natural strengths
- Avoid office politics and social demands that drained her energy

Career Fields That Often Suit AuDHD Women

Research and experience suggest certain career fields tend to be more accommodating for AuDHD traits:

Technology and Engineering: Logical, systematic work with clear parameters and measurable outcomes.

Research and Academia: Opportunities for deep focus, independent work, and specialized expertise.

Creative Fields: Flexibility, variety, and opportunities to hyperfocus on projects of interest.

Healthcare and Helping Professions: Structured environments that benefit from empathy and attention to detail.

Education: Opportunities to share special interests and work in structured environments.

Entrepreneurship: Control over work environment, schedule, and project selection.

The Accommodation-Forward Approach

Rather than hiding their needs, successful AuDHD women often take proactive approaches to workplace accommodations:

Environmental Modifications: Quiet workspaces, adjusted lighting, and sensory accommodations.

Schedule Flexibility: Accommodations for energy fluctuations and optimal performance times.

Communication Preferences: Clear, written instructions and regular feedback cycles.

Project Management: Breaking large projects into smaller, manageable components with clear deadlines.

Case Example: The Accommodation Advocate

Maria transformed her career trajectory by becoming proactive about accommodations:

"I used to struggle through every job, trying to appear normal while constantly overwhelmed. Then I learned about my rights under the ADA and started requesting accommodations upfront. I ask for noise-canceling headphones, written instructions, and flexible start times. Most employers are happy to accommodate when they see the quality of work I produce."

Maria's accommodation requests included:

- A quiet workspace away from high-traffic areas
- Written summaries of verbal instructions
- Flexible scheduling to accommodate energy patterns
- Regular check-ins for feedback and clarification
- Permission to use noise-canceling headphones and other sensory tools

Quarter-Life Crisis Through an AuDHD Lens

The traditional "quarter-life crisis" takes on unique dimensions for AuDHD women, who may experience delayed developmental milestones, extended identity formation, and challenges with traditional life trajectory expectations.

The Delayed Development Reality

AuDHD women often experience what psychologists call "developmental asynchrony"—advanced abilities in some areas coupled with delays in others. This can create confusion and self-doubt during emerging adulthood.

Executive Function Delays: Skills like independent living, financial management, and life planning may lag behind chronological age.

Social Development Variations: Relationship skills and social understanding may develop on different timelines.

Career Readiness Differences: The path to career satisfaction may be longer and more circuitous than for neurotypical peers.

Case Example: The Late Bloomer's Journey

At 25, Rachel felt like she was behind her peers in every area of life:

"My friends were getting married, buying houses, and advancing in their careers. I was still living with roommates, changing majors, and couldn't figure out what I wanted to do with my life. I felt like a failure because I wasn't meeting traditional milestones on schedule."

Rachel's journey illustrates the importance of individualized timelines:

- She didn't graduate college until 24 due to major changes and mental health challenges
- She lived with roommates until 28 while building her freelance career
- She didn't feel ready for serious relationships until her late twenties
- She found career satisfaction through a non-traditional path that honored her neurodivergent needs

Redefining Success Metrics

AuDHD women benefit from developing personalized definitions of success that account for their unique strengths, challenges, and values.

Process Over Outcome Focus: Valuing growth, learning, and effort rather than just achievement.

Authentic Path Recognition: Understanding that their career and life paths may be non-linear and still valid.

Strength-Based Evaluation: Measuring success based on utilizing their natural abilities rather than conforming to external expectations.

Sustainable Lifestyle Prioritization: Valuing mental health, energy management, and authentic relationships over traditional markers of success.

The Identity Integration Process

For many AuDHD women, the twenties involve integrating their neurodivergent identity with their professional and personal aspirations.

From Compensation to Accommodation: Shifting from trying to overcome differences to working with them.

Strength Discovery: Identifying and developing natural abilities rather than focusing solely on deficit areas.

Community Building: Finding others who understand and appreciate neurodivergent perspectives.

Advocacy Development: Learning to advocate for needs and educate others about neurodiversity.

Case Example: The Identity Evolution

Samantha described her identity transformation during her twenties:

"I spent my teens and early twenties trying to be someone I wasn't. I thought success meant acting neurotypical perfectly all the time. But I was exhausted and unfulfilled. My quarter-life crisis was actually an identity crisis—I had to figure out who I really was and what I actually wanted, not what I thought I should want."

Samantha's process involved:

- Therapy focused on self-acceptance and identity development
- Career changes that aligned with her strengths and interests
- Relationship changes that prioritized authenticity over social expectations
- Community involvement in neurodiversity advocacy
- Lifestyle changes that supported her sensory and energy needs

The young adult years for AuDHD women represent a crucial transition period where the foundation for adult success gets established. This phase requires developing sustainable executive function systems, navigating complex relationship dynamics, making career choices that honor neurodivergent strengths, and potentially redefining traditional success metrics.

Success during this period isn't measured by conformity to neurotypical timelines or expectations. Instead, it's defined by the development of self-awareness, authentic relationships, sustainable lifestyle choices, and career paths that utilize natural strengths while accommodating genuine challenges.

AuDHD women who receive appropriate support and develop effective strategies during emerging adulthood are positioned to build fulfilling careers, relationships, and lifestyles that honor their neurodivergent needs while contributing their unique perspectives and abilities to the world.

Moving Forward with Authenticity

The transition through young adulthood with AuDHD requires courage—the courage to be authentic in a world that often rewards conformity, to ask for accommodations in environments that may not understand neurodivergence, and to pursue paths that align with individual strengths and values rather than external expectations.

This foundation of authenticity and self-advocacy becomes increasingly important as AuDHD women face the next major life transition: potential parenthood and the unique challenges of pregnancy and early motherhood with neurodivergent brains.

Core Principles for Young Adult Success

- Executive function management requires external systems and energy-based approaches rather than traditional time management
- Relationship success depends on authentic communication about needs and gradual disclosure strategies
- Career satisfaction comes from environments that accommodate differences while utilizing natural strengths
- Quarter-life challenges may involve delayed developmental timelines that are normal for neurodivergent individuals
- Identity integration during this period creates the foundation for lifelong authenticity and self-advocacy

Chapter 5: Pregnancy and Postpartum

The pregnancy test showed two pink lines at 6 AM on a Thursday morning. Lisa stared at it for a full minute, joy and terror battling in her chest. She'd wanted this baby desperately, had planned for this moment, but as the reality settled in, one thought dominated: How would her AuDHD brain handle the most intense sensory and hormonal experience a human body can undergo?

"I researched everything about pregnancy," Lisa recalled months later, "but nothing prepared me for how my autistic and ADHD traits would interact with pregnancy symptoms. The morning sickness triggered my emetophobia, the hormone surges made my ADHD medication ineffective, and every doctor's appointment felt like sensory torture. I wanted this baby more than anything, but I felt completely unprepared for how pregnancy would affect my neurodivergent brain."

For AuDHD women, pregnancy and postpartum represent the ultimate collision of biological intensity with neurological difference—a time when every system in the body undergoes dramatic change while the brain must adapt to unprecedented demands.

Medication Decisions and Risk Assessment

One of the first and most complex decisions AuDHD women face during pregnancy involves medication management. The choice to continue, modify, or discontinue ADHD medications involves weighing potential risks against the very real consequences of untreated ADHD during pregnancy.

The Medication Discontinuation Reality

Research from ADDitude Magazine reveals that 98% of women discontinue ADHD medications during pregnancy, often based on outdated safety concerns or blanket medical advice that doesn't account for individual risk-benefit analyses.

Case Example: The Executive Function Collapse

Sarah had been managing her AuDHD symptoms successfully with Adderall for five years when she became pregnant. Her obstetrician immediately advised discontinuing the medication, citing potential risks to the baby.

"Within two weeks of stopping my medication, my life fell apart," Sarah remembered. "I couldn't remember prenatal appointments, forgot to take vitamins, and made dangerous mistakes like leaving the stove on. I was having daily meltdowns and couldn't manage basic self-care tasks. The irony was that my inability to function was probably more dangerous to the baby than continuing medication would have been."

Sarah's experience illustrates the complex reality many AuDHD women face: the risks of untreated ADHD during pregnancy may outweigh potential medication risks, especially when considering the mother's ability to engage in healthy pregnancy behaviors.

Current Research on ADHD Medications in Pregnancy

Recent studies provide more nuanced guidance about ADHD medication use during pregnancy:

Stimulant Safety Data: Large-scale studies show that stimulant medications carry relatively low risks when compared to untreated ADHD symptoms.

Functional Impairment Risks: Untreated ADHD increases risks of poor prenatal care adherence, accidents, substance use, and maternal mental health problems.

Individual Risk Assessment: Medical decisions should be based on individual circumstances rather than blanket prohibitions.

The key factors in medication decision-making include:

Severity of ADHD Symptoms: Women with severe functional impairment may benefit from continued medication.

Support System Availability: Women with strong external supports may be better able to manage without medication.

Pregnancy Risks: Individual pregnancy risk factors should be considered alongside ADHD treatment needs.

Alternative Interventions: Non-medication supports like therapy, coaching, and environmental modifications should be maximized.

Case Example: The Collaborative Approach

Maria worked with a maternal-fetal medicine specialist who understood ADHD to develop an individualized plan:

"We looked at my specific situation—I'm a single mom with limited support, I have severe ADHD symptoms that affect my ability to work and care for myself, and I have no other mental health conditions. We decided that staying on a low dose of methylphenidate was safer than going off completely."

Maria's plan included:

- Switching to a shorter-acting stimulant to minimize fetal exposure
- Increasing non-medication supports like executive function coaching
- Regular monitoring of fetal development
- Adjustment of dosing based on changing metabolism during pregnancy
- Clear plans for postpartum medication management

Sensory Overload in New Motherhood

The postpartum period presents unprecedented sensory challenges for AuDHD women. The combination of sleep deprivation, hormonal chaos, and constant infant care creates a perfect storm for sensory overwhelm.

The Sensory Intensity of Newborn Care

Caring for a newborn involves relentless sensory input that can quickly overwhelm AuDHD nervous systems:

Auditory Overwhelm: Crying, especially high-pitched or prolonged crying, can trigger severe stress responses in autistic mothers.

Tactile Overload: Breastfeeding, skin-to-skin contact, and constant physical caregiving can lead to "touched-out" feelings.

Sleep Disruption: The irregular sleep patterns required for newborn care can dysregulate already sensitive nervous systems.

Olfactory Sensitivity: Diaper changes, spit-up, and other infant-related smells can trigger strong aversions.

Case Example: The Breastfeeding Struggle

Amanda had looked forward to breastfeeding but found the experience overwhelming:

"Everyone talks about breastfeeding being this beautiful bonding experience, but for me it was sensory torture. The feeling of the baby latching made my skin crawl. I felt guilty for not enjoying it, which made me question whether I was cut out to be a mother."

Amanda's experience reflects the reality that AuDHD mothers may have different sensory responses to typical caregiving activities. With support from a lactation consultant who understood sensory differences, Amanda developed strategies:

- Using different positioning to minimize uncomfortable sensations
- Implementing sensory breaks between feeding sessions

- Creating a calming environment with dimmed lights and soft music
- Accepting that her breastfeeding experience might look different from others'

Sensory Regulation Strategies for New Mothers

AuDHD mothers need proactive strategies for managing sensory overload during the postpartum period:

Environmental Modifications:

- Creating quiet spaces for recovery between caregiving tasks
- Using noise-canceling headphones when safe to do so
- Adjusting lighting to comfortable levels
- Maintaining comfortable temperatures and textures

Self-Care Prioritization:

- Scheduling regular breaks from sensory-intensive caregiving
- Using compression clothing or weighted blankets for regulation
- Engaging in preferred sensory activities when possible
- Maintaining routines that support nervous system regulation

Support System Activation:

- Asking partners or family members to take over during overwhelm periods
- Communicating specific sensory needs to support people
- Creating backup plans for times when sensory input becomes unmanageable

Case Example: The Regulation Toolkit

Jenny developed a comprehensive sensory regulation toolkit for early motherhood:

"I accepted that I needed more sensory breaks than other mothers, and that was okay. I created a 'sensory rescue kit' with noise-canceling headphones, a soft blanket, peppermint oil for nausea, and fidget toys. When I felt overwhelmed, I'd hand the baby to my partner and take a 10-minute break to regulate."

Jenny's strategies included:

- Pre-planning sensory breaks throughout each day
- Teaching her partner to recognize signs of sensory overwhelm
- Creating sensory-friendly spaces in multiple rooms
- Accepting help with non-essential tasks to preserve energy for caregiving

Distinguishing Postpartum Depression from Autistic Burnout

One of the most critical challenges for AuDHD mothers involves distinguishing between postpartum depression and autistic burnout, as the symptoms can overlap significantly but require different interventions.

Understanding Autistic Burnout

Autistic burnout is a state of physical, mental, and emotional exhaustion caused by prolonged stress and masking. It can occur when autistic individuals exceed their coping capacity for extended periods.

Burnout Symptoms in New Mothers:

- Extreme fatigue that rest doesn't relieve
- Loss of previously developed coping skills
- Increased sensory sensitivities
- Difficulty with basic self-care tasks
- Emotional dysregulation and meltdowns
- Loss of interest in special interests
- Difficulty with executive function tasks

Postpartum Depression Symptoms:

- Persistent sadness or anxiety
- Loss of interest in activities
- Difficulty bonding with the baby
- Thoughts of harming self or baby
- Feelings of guilt or worthlessness
- Changes in appetite or sleep (beyond normal newborn-related disruption)

The Overlap Challenge

Many symptoms appear in both conditions, making differential diagnosis challenging:

Fatigue: Both conditions involve extreme tiredness, but burnout fatigue often feels different from depression fatigue.

Emotional Dysregulation: Both can involve mood swings and emotional intensity.

Functional Impairment: Both conditions can interfere with daily functioning and caregiving abilities.

Social Withdrawal: Both may lead to isolation and difficulty maintaining relationships.

Case Example: The Misdiagnosis Journey

Rebecca was diagnosed with postpartum depression at 6 weeks postpartum, but antidepressant medication didn't help her symptoms:

"The psychiatrist kept increasing my antidepressant dose, but I felt worse, not better. I was exhausted all the time, couldn't handle any sensory input, and felt like I'd lost all my coping skills. It wasn't until I started working with a therapist who understood autism that we realized I was experiencing burnout, not depression."

Rebecca's recovery involved:

- Reducing sensory input and social demands
- Rebuilding basic self-care routines
- Gradually reintroducing previously helpful coping strategies
- Addressing the underlying causes of burnout rather than just symptoms
- Developing sustainable approaches to motherhood that honored her autistic needs

Integrated Assessment Approaches

Effective evaluation requires understanding both conditions and their potential interaction:

Comprehensive History: Examining pre-pregnancy functioning, previous episodes of burnout or depression, and family history.

Symptom Timeline: Understanding when symptoms began and how they've changed over time.

Response to Interventions: Monitoring how symptoms respond to different types of support and treatment.

Contextual Factors: Considering life stressors, support availability, and environmental factors.

Case Example: The Dual Diagnosis Reality

Some women experience both postpartum depression and autistic burnout simultaneously:

Lisa's evaluation revealed that she was experiencing both conditions: "I had legitimate postpartum depression that responded well to medication and therapy. But I also had autistic burnout from the overwhelming demands of new motherhood. I needed treatment for both—antidepressants for the depression and sensory accommodations plus stress reduction for the burnout."

Building Comprehensive Support Systems

AuDHD mothers need support systems that understand both their neurodivergent needs and the challenges of new parenthood. Effective support addresses practical needs, emotional well-being, and sensory regulation.

The Multi-Layered Support Approach

Comprehensive support for AuDHD mothers involves multiple types of assistance:

Practical Support: Help with household tasks, meal preparation, and basic life management during the overwhelming early weeks.

Emotional Support: Understanding and validation from people who recognize the unique challenges of neurodivergent motherhood.

Professional Support: Healthcare providers, therapists, and coaches who understand both postpartum challenges and neurodivergent presentations.

Peer Support: Connection with other neurodivergent mothers who can provide understanding and practical strategies.

Case Example: The Village Approach

Sarah assembled what she called her "neurodivergent village":

"I realized I needed different types of support from different people. My mom handled practical stuff like meals and laundry. My neurodivergent friends provided emotional understanding. My therapist helped with mental health. My postpartum doula understood both birth recovery and sensory needs."

Sarah's support network included:

- Family members who handled household management

- A postpartum doula trained in neurodivergent needs
- A therapist specializing in maternal mental health and autism
- Online communities of neurodivergent mothers
- A few close friends who understood her sensory and energy needs

Partner Education and Support

Partners play crucial roles in supporting AuDHD mothers but often need education about neurodivergent presentations and needs:

Understanding Sensory Differences: Learning to recognize and respond to sensory overwhelm.

Supporting Regulation: Knowing how to help with nervous system regulation and recovery.

Sharing Caregiving: Taking on infant care during overwhelming periods.

Advocating with Professionals: Supporting accurate diagnosis and appropriate treatment.

Case Example: The Learning Partnership

Mark initially struggled to understand his partner's postpartum experience:

"I didn't understand why routine doctor visits sent her into meltdowns or why she needed so many breaks from holding the baby. I thought she just wasn't bonding properly. Once I learned about sensory processing and autistic burnout, I could see what was really happening and provide better support."

Mark's education involved:

- Reading about autism and ADHD in women
- Attending therapy sessions to understand his partner's needs

- Learning to recognize signs of sensory overload
- Developing practical strategies for sharing caregiving responsibilities
- Advocating with healthcare providers who didn't understand neurodivergent presentations

Professional Support Considerations

AuDHD mothers need healthcare providers who understand both postpartum experiences and neurodivergent presentations:

Screening Adaptations: Using assessment tools that account for neurodivergent presentations.

Treatment Modifications: Adapting interventions for sensory sensitivities and executive function differences.

Integrated Care: Coordinating between different providers to address multiple needs.

Long-term Perspective: Understanding that recovery may take longer and look different for neurodivergent mothers.

The Acceptance and Accommodation Approach

Successful support for AuDHD mothers involves accepting that their experience may be different from neurotypical mothers and providing appropriate accommodations:

Different Timeline Expectations: Understanding that adjustment to motherhood may take longer.

Modified Bonding Expectations: Recognizing that bonding may happen differently and still be valid.

Sensory Accommodation: Providing environments and experiences that support rather than overwhelm.

Strength-Based Focus: Emphasizing the unique strengths AuDHD mothers bring to parenting.

Case Example: The Strength Discovery

Emma initially felt like she was failing at motherhood until she reframed her experience:

"I thought I was a terrible mother because I couldn't handle baby groups, needed so many breaks, and found breastfeeding overwhelming. But my therapist helped me see my strengths—I'm incredibly attentive to my baby's subtle cues, I create predictable routines that help him feel secure, and my attention to detail means I notice things other parents miss."

Emma's strengths included:

- Exceptional observation skills that helped her understand her baby's needs
- Ability to create structured routines that benefited infant development
- Attention to detail that supported health and safety
- Deep empathy that fostered secure attachment once sensory challenges were managed

Pregnancy and postpartum with AuDHD requires a fundamental shift from trying to have a "normal" experience to creating an experience that works for neurodivergent brains and bodies. This involves making informed decisions about medication, developing strategies for managing sensory overload, accurately identifying and treating mental health challenges, and building support systems that understand and accommodate neurodivergent needs.

Success during this period isn't measured by conformity to typical pregnancy and postpartum experiences. Instead, it's defined by healthy outcomes for both mother and baby, sustainable coping strategies, and the development of parenting approaches that honor neurodivergent strengths while managing genuine challenges.

AuDHD mothers who receive appropriate support and develop effective strategies during pregnancy and postpartum are positioned to build fulfilling relationships with their children while maintaining their own well-being and authentic identity.

Looking Toward Future Challenges

The experience of pregnancy and early motherhood with AuDHD provides important lessons about managing neurological differences during times of intense biological and social change. These skills become increasingly important as women face the next major hormonal transition: perimenopause and the unique challenges it presents for AuDHD brains.

Core Elements for Success in AuDHD Motherhood

- Medication decisions require individual risk-benefit analysis rather than blanket prohibitions
- Sensory overload management is essential for successful adjustment to motherhood
- Accurate diagnosis distinguishing postpartum depression from autistic burnout is crucial for appropriate treatment
- Comprehensive support systems must address practical, emotional, and professional needs
- Acceptance of different experiences and timelines supports authentic, successful motherhood

Chapter 6: Perimenopause - The Storm Before the Calm

The email sat in Dr. Martinez's inbox for three days before she could bring herself to open it. The subject line read "Help - I think I'm losing my mind," and the sender was Patricia, one of her most accomplished patients—a 47-year-old executive who had managed her AuDHD symptoms successfully for decades.

"Dr. Martinez," the email began, "I don't know what's happening to me. For 20 years, I've had systems and routines that worked. I could handle my job, maintain my relationships, and manage my symptoms. But over the past six months, everything has fallen apart. I can't concentrate in meetings I used to lead confidently. Sounds that never bothered me are unbearable. I'm having meltdowns over things that wouldn't have fazed me before. My husband thinks I'm having a breakdown, and honestly, so do I."

Patricia was experiencing perimenopause—the hormonal transition that researchers and AuDHD women themselves describe as potentially the most challenging phase of their lives.

Why This Phase Is "Most Challenging" for AuDHD

Research from ADDitude Magazine confirms what many AuDHD women experience firsthand: perimenopause represents a perfect storm of neurological and hormonal changes that can destabilize even the most sophisticated coping systems developed over decades.

The Hormonal Chaos of Perimenopause

Unlike the gradual hormonal decline once believed to characterize menopause, recent research reveals that perimenopause involves dramatic, unpredictable fluctuations that can occur over 4-10 years. For AuDHD women, whose brains are already sensitive to neurochemical changes, these fluctuations create unprecedented challenges.

Estrogen's Erratic Dance: During perimenopause, estrogen levels don't decline smoothly but instead swing wildly—sometimes reaching higher levels than during reproductive years, then plummeting to menopausal levels within days or weeks.

Progesterone's Early Exit: Progesterone often declines before estrogen, disrupting the delicate balance between these hormones and affecting sleep, mood, and cognitive function.

Unpredictable Patterns: The monthly cycles that many AuDHD women relied on for symptom prediction become irregular and unreliable.

Case Example: The Executive's Crisis

Patricia had spent two decades developing what she called her "symptom management system":

"I knew exactly when my ADHD symptoms would be worse each month. I scheduled important meetings during my high-functioning weeks and built in recovery time during difficult periods. I had systems for everything—meal planning, work organization, social obligations. But perimenopause destroyed all my predictability."

Patricia's experience illustrates how perimenopause can undermine previously effective strategies:

- Her reliable monthly patterns disappeared, making symptom prediction impossible
- Previously effective medications became inconsistent in their effects
- Sensory sensitivities that had been manageable became overwhelming
- Executive function systems that worked for decades suddenly felt inadequate
- Social situations she'd mastered became anxiety-provoking again

The Amplification Effect

61

Perimenopause doesn't just add new symptoms—it amplifies existing AuDHD traits in ways that can feel overwhelming:

Sensory Sensitivity Intensification: Sounds, textures, lights, and smells that were manageable become unbearable.

Executive Function Breakdown: Organizational systems that worked for years become inadequate for the increased cognitive demands.

Emotional Dysregulation Escalation: The emotional intensity characteristic of ADHD becomes more extreme and harder to manage.

Masking Fatigue: The energy required to maintain social masks becomes unsustainable.

Research Findings on Perimenopause and AuDHD

A comprehensive ADDitude survey of over 1,500 women revealed striking findings about perimenopause's impact on AuDHD symptoms:

94% of women reported that their ADHD symptoms grew more severe during perimenopause and menopause.

70% experienced "life-altering impact" from brain fog and overwhelm during their 40s and 50s, compared to only 11% who reported similar impact in their 20s and 30s.

Memory and cognitive problems became the most debilitating symptoms, with many women fearing early-onset dementia.

Case Example: The Misdiagnosed Crisis

Jennifer, a 49-year-old teacher, sought medical help when her symptoms became unmanageable:

"My doctor ran every test imaginable—thyroid, vitamin levels, MRI scans. Everything came back normal, so he suggested antidepressants. But I wasn't depressed—I was cognitively impaired. I couldn't remember my students' names, lost track of conversations mid-sentence, and couldn't follow lesson plans I'd taught for years."

Jennifer's experience reflects a common pattern: healthcare providers often miss the connection between perimenopause and AuDHD symptom intensification, leading to inappropriate treatments and prolonged suffering.

Managing Symptom Intensification

The key to managing perimenopause with AuDHD lies in understanding that this isn't a personal failure or loss of coping skills—it's a neurobiological response to dramatic hormonal changes that requires adapted strategies.

Symptom Tracking and Pattern Recognition

While monthly patterns become unreliable during perimenopause, tracking can still reveal useful information:

Expanded Tracking Variables:

- Daily symptom severity across multiple domains
- Sleep quality and patterns
- Stress levels and triggers
- Physical symptoms like hot flashes and fatigue
- Cognitive function indicators
- Medication effectiveness

Weekly and Monthly Pattern Analysis: Look for patterns across longer timeframes since daily cycles become less predictable.

Trigger Identification: Focus on identifying environmental, social, and physical triggers that worsen symptoms.

Case Example: The Data-Driven Approach

Maria, a 45-year-old researcher, applied her analytical skills to understanding her perimenopause experience:

"I tracked everything for six months—symptoms, sleep, stress, weather, work demands, social obligations. I discovered that while my monthly patterns were gone, I still had some predictability. High-stress weeks were always followed by symptom flares. Social overcommitment led to sensory overwhelm. Understanding these patterns helped me make adjustments."

Maria's insights led to practical changes:

- Scheduling recovery time after high-stress periods
- Limiting social commitments during weeks with work deadlines
- Adjusting medication timing based on sleep patterns rather than menstrual cycles
- Creating flexible backup plans for days when symptoms were severe

Adaptive Coping Strategies

Perimenopause requires more flexible, adaptive approaches than the rigid systems that may have worked during reproductive years:

The Buffer Strategy: Building extra time, energy, and resources into all plans to accommodate unpredictable symptom fluctuations.

Multiple System Backups: Developing several different approaches to important tasks so that alternatives exist when primary systems fail.

Energy Conservation: Prioritizing essential activities and eliminating non-critical demands during difficult periods.

Professional Support Intensification: Increasing therapeutic, medical, and practical support during this challenging transition.

Medication Adjustments and Hormone Therapy

The hormonal chaos of perimenopause often requires significant adjustments to both ADHD medications and consideration of hormone replacement therapy.

ADHD Medication Challenges in Perimenopause

Many women find that ADHD medications that worked consistently for years become unpredictable during perimenopause:

Effectiveness Fluctuations: Medications may work well some days and poorly others, corresponding to hormonal changes.

Dosage Inadequacy: Previously effective doses may become insufficient during low-estrogen phases.

Side Effect Changes: Women may experience new or intensified side effects as their hormone levels change.

Case Example: The Medication Roller Coaster

Susan had taken the same dose of Adderall for eight years with consistent results. At 46, her experience changed dramatically:

"Some days, my medication worked perfectly. Other days, it felt like I'd taken nothing at all. My doctor suggested increasing the dose, but that led to anxiety and sleep problems. We realized the issue wasn't the medication itself but how my changing hormones affected its absorption and effectiveness."

Susan's solution involved:

- Working with a psychiatrist experienced in hormonal influences on ADHD
- Adjusting dosing strategies rather than just increasing overall amounts
- Adding short-acting medications for breakthrough symptoms

- Timing doses to correspond with predicted low-estrogen periods
- Monitoring and adjusting based on hormonal patterns rather than fixed schedules

Hormone Replacement Therapy Considerations

Research suggests that hormone replacement therapy (HRT) can significantly benefit AuDHD women during perimenopause by stabilizing the hormonal fluctuations that worsen symptoms.

HRT Benefits for AuDHD Women:

- Improved cognitive function and memory
- Reduced sensory sensitivities
- Better emotional regulation
- Enhanced ADHD medication effectiveness
- Improved sleep quality

Types of HRT for AuDHD Women:

Estrogen Replacement: Can improve dopamine function and reduce ADHD symptoms.

Progesterone Addition: May help with sleep and anxiety but can sometimes worsen ADHD symptoms.

Testosterone Consideration: Some women benefit from small amounts of testosterone for energy and cognitive function.

Delivery Methods: Patches, gels, and other transdermal methods may provide more stable hormone levels than oral medications.

Case Example: The HRT Success Story

After struggling for two years with worsening symptoms, Lisa decided to try hormone replacement therapy:

"Within six weeks of starting estrogen patches, I felt like myself again. My brain fog lifted, my ADHD medication started working consistently, and I could handle sensory input that had been overwhelming me. It wasn't a complete solution, but it gave me back the stability I needed to use my other coping strategies."

Lisa's HRT regimen included:

- Estradiol patches for steady hormone delivery
- Micronized progesterone for sleep and mood support
- Regular monitoring of hormone levels and symptom response
- Coordination with her ADHD medication prescriber
- Lifestyle modifications to support hormonal balance

Integrated Treatment Approaches

The most successful perimenopause management often involves coordinating multiple interventions:

Medical Team Coordination: Working with gynecologists, psychiatrists, and primary care providers who communicate about treatment approaches.

Timing Strategies: Coordinating ADHD medication adjustments with HRT initiation for optimal results.

Monitoring Protocols: Regular assessment of both ADHD symptoms and menopausal symptoms to guide treatment decisions.

Lifestyle Integration: Combining medical treatments with dietary, exercise, and stress management approaches.

Mental Health Protection Strategies

Perimenopause significantly increases the risk of depression, anxiety, and other mental health challenges for all women, but AuDHD women face additional vulnerabilities that require proactive protection strategies.

Understanding Increased Mental Health Risks

Several factors contribute to heightened mental health risks during perimenopause for AuDHD women:

Hormonal Vulnerability: The same hormonal fluctuations that worsen ADHD and autism symptoms also increase depression and anxiety risk.

Coping System Breakdown: When established coping mechanisms become ineffective, stress and mental health symptoms often increase.

Identity Disruption: Feeling like a different person or losing capabilities can trigger existential distress.

Social Isolation: Increased sensory sensitivities and social fatigue can lead to withdrawal and loneliness.

Case Example: The Spiral Prevention

Rebecca recognized early warning signs and took proactive steps:

"I noticed I was starting to avoid social situations I used to handle fine and was having trouble completing work tasks that were usually routine. Instead of waiting for things to get worse, I immediately increased my therapy sessions, started a support group, and talked to my psychiatrist about medication adjustments."

Rebecca's prevention strategy included:

- Weekly therapy sessions focused on coping strategy adaptation
- Joining a perimenopause support group for women with ADHD
- Meditation and mindfulness practices adapted for ADHD brains
- Regular psychiatric monitoring and medication adjustments
- Social connection maintenance through low-demand activities

Building Emotional Resilience

Effective mental health protection during perimenopause involves building resilience before crisis points:

Therapeutic Support: Regular therapy focused on adaptation strategies and emotional processing.

Peer Connection: Relationships with other AuDHD women navigating similar challenges.

Identity Work: Developing self-worth that isn't dependent on consistent performance or capability.

Stress Management: Techniques specifically adapted for neurodivergent brains and sensory sensitivities.

The Self-Compassion Imperative

Perhaps the most crucial mental health protection strategy involves developing radical self-compassion during this challenging transition:

Normalizing the Experience: Understanding that perimenopause difficulties are neurobiological, not personal failures.

Adjusting Expectations: Accepting that this phase may require reduced demands and increased support.

Celebrating Adaptation: Recognizing the strength it takes to navigate these challenges and develop new coping strategies.

Future Focus: Maintaining hope that this is a transition phase, not a permanent deterioration.

Case Example: The Compassion Transformation

At 48, Diana learned to extend herself the compassion she'd always given others:

"I spent the first year of perimenopause berating myself for not being able to handle things I'd managed easily before. Then I realized I was expecting myself to function normally during what amounts to major neurological chaos. I started treating myself with the same kindness I'd show a friend going through this experience."

Diana's self-compassion practice included:

- Daily self-talk monitoring and correction
- Permission to have bad days without shame
- Celebration of small victories and adaptations
- Boundary setting that prioritized her well-being
- Advocacy for understanding from family and colleagues

Professional Mental Health Support

AuDHD women benefit from mental health providers who understand both perimenopausal challenges and neurodivergent presentations:

Specialized Knowledge: Therapists who understand how hormonal changes affect neurodivergent brains.

Integrated Approaches: Treatment that addresses hormonal, neurological, and psychological factors simultaneously.

Adaptation Focus: Therapy focused on developing new strategies rather than just managing symptoms.

Long-term Perspective: Understanding that perimenopause is a transition requiring sustained support.

Perimenopause with AuDHD represents one of the most challenging transitions many women will face, but it's also temporary. The key to successful navigation lies in understanding that this isn't a personal failure or permanent decline—it's a neurobiological response to dramatic hormonal changes that requires adapted strategies, increased support, and tremendous self-compassion.

Women who receive appropriate medical care, develop flexible coping strategies, and maintain strong support systems can not only survive perimenopause but emerge with deeper self-knowledge, improved advocacy skills, and more sustainable approaches to managing their AuDHD traits.

The experience of navigating perimenopause successfully provides valuable preparation for the next phase: menopause and beyond, where many women discover unexpected benefits and opportunities for authentic living.

The Light at the End of the Tunnel

While perimenopause may be the storm, it's important to remember that it's the storm before the calm. Many AuDHD women find that post-menopausal life, while different from their reproductive years, offers unique opportunities for authenticity, reduced hormonal chaos, and the application of hard-won wisdom about managing their neurodivergent traits.

Essential Survival Strategies for the Perimenopausal Storm

- Recognize that symptom intensification is neurobiological, not personal failure
- Develop flexible, adaptive coping systems that can accommodate unpredictable fluctuations
- Consider coordinated medical interventions including ADHD medication adjustments and hormone therapy
- Prioritize mental health protection through increased support and radical self-compassion
- Maintain hope that this challenging transition leads to greater stability and self-knowledge

Chapter 7: Menopause and Beyond - Finding Your New Normal

The hot flash hit at exactly 10:43 AM during the quarterly board meeting, but for the first time in two years, Margaret didn't panic. At 54, she'd been post-menopausal for eight months, and something unexpected was happening—she was starting to feel more like herself than she had in decades.

"I spent my forties feeling like I was losing my mind," Margaret reflected. "Perimenopause was brutal. But now that my hormones have settled into their new pattern, I'm discovering things about myself I never knew. I'm less anxious about social situations, more confident in my opinions, and somehow more comfortable being authentically me."

Margaret's experience reflects a surprising reality that many AuDHD women discover: while the transition through perimenopause is challenging, post-menopausal life can offer unexpected benefits and opportunities for authentic living that were harder to access during the hormonal chaos of reproductive years.

Unexpected Benefits of Post-Menopausal AuDHD

Research and lived experience reveal that many AuDHD women find post-menopausal life surprisingly liberating. The stabilization of hormone levels, combined with reduced social pressures and increased self-knowledge, creates opportunities for authentic expression that may have been suppressed for decades.

Hormonal Stability and Cognitive Clarity

While the dramatic estrogen fluctuations of perimenopause intensify AuDHD symptoms, the stable (though lower) hormone levels of post-menopause can actually provide relief for some women.

Predictable Patterns: Without monthly hormonal fluctuations, many women find their symptoms become more predictable and manageable.

Reduced Emotional Intensity: The emotional volatility associated with hormonal fluctuations often stabilizes, making emotional regulation easier.

Clearer Thinking: The brain fog of perimenopause frequently lifts, revealing clearer cognitive function.

Case Example: The Stability Discovery

Sharon, 56, had struggled with ADHD symptom variability for decades:

"My entire adult life, I never knew which version of myself I'd wake up as. Some days I was sharp and focused, others I could barely function. Post-menopause, I finally have consistency. My ADHD symptoms are still there, but they're predictable. I can plan around them instead of being surprised by them every month."

Sharon's post-menopausal experience included:

- Consistent response to ADHD medications without monthly fluctuations
- Stable energy patterns that allowed for better life planning
- Reduced sensory sensitivity compared to perimenopausal peaks
- More consistent sleep patterns leading to better overall functioning

The Masking Reduction Phenomenon

Many AuDHD women report that post-menopause brings a natural reduction in the urge to mask autistic traits, leading to greater authenticity and reduced exhaustion.

Decreased Social Pressure: Post-menopausal women often face fewer social expectations about appearance, behavior, and performance.

Increased Self-Acceptance: Decades of life experience often lead to greater self-acceptance and reduced need for external validation.

Energy Conservation: Without the metabolic demands of reproductive hormones, many women have more energy available for authentic expression rather than masking.

Case Example: The Unmasking Journey

Linda, 58, described her post-menopausal transformation:

"I spent my entire adult life trying to appear 'normal'—forcing eye contact, suppressing my stims, pretending to enjoy social events I found draining. After menopause, something shifted. I stopped caring so much about what others thought and started honoring what I actually needed. I use my fidget toys openly now, I leave parties when I'm tired, and I talk about my interests without apologizing."

Linda's changes included:

- Open stimming in public without shame
- Honest communication about sensory needs
- Pursuit of special interests without embarrassment
- Boundary setting that prioritized her well-being
- Authentic expression of her autistic traits in social settings

Enhanced Focus on Special Interests

Without the demands of reproductive hormones and often with increased time due to life stage changes, many AuDHD women find post-menopause ideal for pursuing special interests with unprecedented depth.

Increased Available Energy: Without monthly hormonal energy drains, more resources become available for focused pursuits.

Reduced External Obligations: Changes in family responsibilities often create more time for personal interests.

Decreased Social Pressure: Less pressure to engage in socially expected activities creates space for authentic pursuits.

Case Example: The Artist's Renaissance

Patricia, 61, experienced what she called her "artistic renaissance":

"I'd always been interested in painting but never had the sustained focus or energy to develop real skill. Post-menopause, I finally had the consistency and freedom to hyperfocus on art. I've produced more meaningful work in the past five years than in the previous thirty. My ADHD hyperfocus, which used to be scattered across a dozen interests, finally had the stability to sustain long-term projects."

Patricia's artistic development included:

- Daily painting practice enabled by stable energy patterns
- Deep study of techniques that engaged her systematic thinking
- Gallery shows that celebrated her unique perspective
- Art teaching that combined her interests with helping others
- Community connections through art groups that provided social connection without masking demands

Redefining Productivity and Success Metrics

Post-menopausal life offers AuDHD women the opportunity to fundamentally redefine what productivity and success mean, moving away from externally imposed standards toward personally meaningful metrics.

Moving Beyond Traditional Productivity

The conventional productivity model—consistent output, multitasking ability, and neurotypical work patterns—often becomes less relevant as AuDHD women age and gain self-knowledge.

Quality Over Quantity Focus: Many women discover that their deep-focus abilities produce higher-quality results when they stop trying to match neurotypical productivity patterns.

Energy-Based Achievement: Success becomes measured by energy management and sustainable practices rather than raw output.

Authentic Contribution: Focus shifts to making meaningful contributions that align with personal values and strengths.

Case Example: The Consultant's Revolution

Maria, 55, transformed her career approach after menopause:

"I spent twenty years trying to be the kind of consultant who could handle multiple clients, constant networking, and back-to-back meetings. I was successful by conventional metrics but exhausted and unfulfilled. Post-menopause, I restructured everything. Now I work with fewer clients but provide much deeper, more valuable services. My income actually increased because I'm working with my AuDHD strengths instead of against them."

Maria's business transformation included:

- Reducing client load to allow for deeper focus on each project
- Scheduling intensive work periods with built-in recovery time
- Specializing in areas that utilized her systematic thinking and attention to detail
- Creating sensory-friendly work environments that supported her best performance
- Marketing her neurodivergent perspective as a unique value proposition

The Sustainability Revolution

Post-menopausal AuDHD women often develop sophisticated understanding of sustainability—what can be maintained long-term without causing burnout or health problems.

Energy Budget Management: Treating energy as a finite resource that must be allocated thoughtfully.

Seasonal Approaches: Adapting activities and commitments to natural rhythms and capacity fluctuations.

Recovery Integration: Building rest and restoration into all plans rather than treating them as luxuries.

Boundary Sophistication: Developing nuanced understanding of when to say yes and when to decline opportunities.

Case Example: The Teacher's Wisdom

Janet, 59, revolutionized her approach to teaching after menopause:

"I used to say yes to every committee, every extra duty, every social obligation at work. I thought that's what good teachers did. After menopause, I realized I could be a much better teacher if I focused my energy on what I did best—creating innovative curricula and supporting struggling students—rather than trying to do everything. My students benefit more from my focused attention than they ever did from my scattered efforts."

Janet's sustainable teaching practice included:

- Selective committee participation based on genuine interest and expertise
- Classroom modifications that supported both her needs and student learning
- Professional development focused on her strengths rather than deficit areas
- Collaboration with colleagues that played to everyone's strengths
- Work-life boundaries that preserved energy for quality teaching

Late Diagnosis Revelations and Identity Integration

Many AuDHD women receive their first diagnosis during menopause or post-menopause, creating unique opportunities and challenges for identity integration later in life.

The Late Diagnosis Phenomenon

Several factors contribute to increased AuDHD diagnosis rates among menopausal and post-menopausal women:

Symptom Unmasking: Hormonal changes and reduced masking reveal previously hidden traits.

Advocacy Increase: Greater awareness and advocacy around women's neurodivergence creates more diagnostic opportunities.

Life Stage Reflection: Major life transitions often prompt self-examination and help-seeking.

Family Connections: Many women seek evaluation after their children are diagnosed.

Case Example: The 52-Year-Old Student

Dorothy received her AuDHD diagnosis at 52, after struggling through perimenopause:

"Everything finally made sense. The social exhaustion I'd felt my whole life, the sensory issues I thought everyone had, the way I needed so much more structure than other people—it all had an explanation. I wasn't defective or weak; I was neurodivergent. It was overwhelming and liberating at the same time."

Dorothy's diagnostic journey included:

- Initial evaluation prompted by her daughter's autism diagnosis
- Recognition of lifelong patterns she'd attributed to personality quirks
- Relief at finally having explanations for decades of struggles

- Grief for the woman she might have been with earlier support
- Excitement about applying new self-knowledge to her remaining years

The Identity Reconstruction Process

Late diagnosis requires reconstructing decades of self-understanding and life narrative through a neurodivergent lens.

Life Story Reframing: Understanding past experiences as neurodivergent responses rather than personal failures.

Relationship Reevaluation: Examining relationships and social patterns through the lens of autism and ADHD.

Career Reflection: Understanding professional challenges and successes in terms of neurodivergent traits.

Future Planning: Making life decisions based on authentic self-knowledge rather than assumed neurotypical needs.

Case Example: The Marketing Executive's Rewrite

Sylvia, diagnosed at 58, spent months reexamining her life story:

"I always thought I was just antisocial, disorganized, and too sensitive. Looking back through my AuDHD diagnosis, I could see patterns everywhere. The jobs I loved were the ones that matched my hyperfocus abilities. The relationships that worked were with people who accepted my directness and need for routine. The social situations I avoided were actually sensory nightmares. Understanding this gave me a roadmap for making better choices going forward."

Sylvia's reframing process involved:

- Journaling about past experiences with new understanding
- Therapy focused on identity integration and self-acceptance

- Conversations with family members about newly understood behaviors
- Career pivots that better aligned with her neurodivergent strengths
- Social life restructuring around authentic preferences and needs

The Grief and Celebration Balance

Late diagnosis often involves simultaneous grief for past struggles and celebration of new understanding.

Mourning the Misunderstood Past: Grieving years of unnecessary struggle and self-criticism.

Celebrating Current Insights: Joy at finally understanding oneself and having explanations for lifelong patterns.

Anger at Systems: Frustration with medical and educational systems that missed obvious signs.

Hope for the Future: Excitement about living authentically with proper support and accommodations.

Creating Meaningful Second Acts

Post-menopausal life offers AuDHD women opportunities to create what many call "second acts"—new chapters focused on authentic expression, meaningful contribution, and sustainable practices.

The Freedom to Authenticity

Many post-menopausal AuDHD women describe feeling freed from social expectations that constrained their earlier years.

Reduced Performance Pressure: Less pressure to conform to conventional expectations of femininity, productivity, and social behavior.

Increased Self-Knowledge: Decades of experience provide clear understanding of strengths, preferences, and needs.

Enhanced Advocacy Skills: Years of navigating challenges create sophisticated self-advocacy abilities.

Case Example: The Nonprofit Founder

Rachel, 64, launched her dream organization at 60:

"I spent my career in corporate environments that demanded constant masking and performance. After menopause, I realized I had maybe twenty good years left—I wasn't going to waste them pretending to be someone I wasn't. I started a nonprofit supporting neurodivergent adults, work that uses every aspect of my AuDHD traits as strengths."

Rachel's second act included:

- Organization focused on her lifelong passion for helping neurodivergent individuals
- Work environment designed around her sensory and social needs
- Team structure that leveraged her systematic thinking and attention to detail
- Public speaking that celebrated rather than hid her autistic directness
- Legacy building that gave deep meaning to her remaining working years

Contribution Through Difference

Many AuDHD women find that their neurodivergent perspectives become valuable contributions in their post-menopausal years.

Unique Viewpoints: Lifelong experience as outsiders provides valuable perspectives on systems and solutions.

Deep Expertise: Years of hyperfocus on special interests create genuine expertise that can benefit others.

Empathy and Understanding: Personal experience with struggle creates exceptional ability to help others facing similar challenges.

Case Example: The Therapist's Specialization

Linda, 57, developed a thriving practice specializing in late-diagnosed neurodivergent women:

"My own diagnostic journey at 54 gave me insights no textbook could provide. I understand the shame, confusion, and relief my clients experience because I've lived it. My AuDHD traits—my attention to detail, my systematic approach to therapy, my direct communication style—are exactly what these women need."

Linda's specialized practice included:

- Client base composed entirely of women seeking late diagnosis or post-diagnosis support
- Therapy approaches adapted for neurodivergent minds and sensory sensitivities
- Group programs that provided community and understanding
- Advocacy work with medical providers about recognizing AuDHD in older women
- Training programs for other therapists working with neurodivergent adults

The Mentorship Opportunity

Post-menopausal AuDHD women often become valuable mentors for younger neurodivergent individuals navigating similar challenges.

Lived Experience Wisdom: Decades of navigating neurodivergent life provide practical wisdom younger people desperately need.

Perspective on Challenges: Understanding that current difficulties are often temporary and manageable.

Model of Possibilities: Demonstrating that neurodivergent women can build fulfilling, authentic lives.

Case Example: The Community Builder

Margaret, 61, became a community organizer for neurodivergent women:

"I wish I'd had older neurodivergent women to look up to when I was struggling through my twenties and thirties. Now I try to be that person for younger women. I share my story, offer practical advice, and mostly just show them that it's possible to build a good life as an AuDHD woman."

Margaret's community work included:

- Monthly support groups for neurodivergent women of all ages
- Mentorship programs pairing older and younger neurodivergent women
- Workshops on practical life skills adapted for AuDHD needs
- Advocacy efforts focused on improving services for neurodivergent adults
- Social events designed to be sensory-friendly and authentic

The Creative Renaissance

Many AuDHD women experience creative flourishing in their post-menopausal years as they gain time, stability, and freedom to pursue authentic interests.

Uninterrupted Focus: Freedom from hormonal chaos and many external obligations allows for sustained creative work.

Authentic Expression: Reduced need for masking enables more genuine creative expression.

Resource Availability: Often increased financial stability and life experience provide resources for creative pursuits.

Case Example: The Writer's Victory

Susan, 59, published her first novel at 58:

"I'd been writing secretly for decades but never thought my work was good enough to share. After menopause, I stopped caring about perfect prose and started caring about authentic stories. My novel about a late-diagnosed autistic woman resonated with readers because it came from genuine experience, not textbook knowledge."

Susan's creative journey included:

- Daily writing practice enabled by stable post-menopausal routines
- Stories that celebrated neurodivergent perspectives rather than hiding them
- Publishing success that validated her unique voice and experiences
- Speaking engagements that combined her interests in writing and neurodiversity advocacy
- Community building with other neurodivergent creative professionals

Building Legacy and Meaning

Post-menopausal AuDHD women often focus on creating lasting impact and meaning, using their accumulated wisdom and authentic self-knowledge to benefit others and contribute to positive change.

The Advocacy Evolution

Many women who spent years advocating for themselves begin advocating for broader systemic change.

System Change Focus: Working to improve diagnosis, services, and understanding for future generations of neurodivergent women.

Professional Influence: Using career positions to create more inclusive, neurodiversity-friendly environments.

Community Leadership: Taking leadership roles in neurodiversity organizations and advocacy groups.

Case Example: The Doctor's Mission

Dr. Patricia Williams, diagnosed with AuDHD at 55, transformed her medical practice:

"Once I understood my own neurodivergence, I couldn't unsee it in my patients. I began screening more systematically for autism and ADHD in women, especially during major hormonal transitions. I've diagnosed dozens of women who had been missed by the system for decades. It's become my professional mission."

Dr. Williams' advocacy work included:

- Protocol development for screening AuDHD in women during menopause
- Training programs for other healthcare providers
- Research participation in studies of neurodivergence in aging women
- Medical journal articles about hormonal influences on AuDHD symptoms
- Conference presentations sharing her professional and personal insights

The post-menopausal years for AuDHD women represent a unique opportunity for authentic living, meaningful contribution, and sustainable success. The combination of hormonal stability, reduced social pressures, increased self-knowledge, and often greater life resources creates conditions for flourishing that may not have been possible during earlier life stages.

This phase isn't about declining abilities or reduced potential—it's about finally having the stability, wisdom, and freedom to live authentically and contribute meaningfully. Many AuDHD women find their post-menopausal years to be their most fulfilling, creative, and impactful period of life.

The journey through hormonal chaos to post-menopausal stability provides valuable lessons about resilience, adaptation, and the importance of authentic self-knowledge. These women become living examples that neurodivergent life can be not just manageable but truly flourishing.

The Wisdom Integration

The experience of navigating AuDHD through all life stages—from the hidden struggles of youth through the hormonal storms of midlife to the authentic flowering of post-menopause—creates a unique form of wisdom. This wisdom combines deep self-knowledge with practical strategies, systemic understanding with personal resilience, and individual growth with community contribution.

Post-menopausal AuDHD women who have successfully navigated these transitions become invaluable resources for younger generations, healthcare providers, and society as a whole. They demonstrate that neurodivergent life paths, while different from conventional expectations, can lead to profound fulfillment, meaningful contribution, and authentic success.

Essential Elements for Post-Menopausal Flourishing

- Hormonal stability can provide unprecedented consistency and predictability for AuDHD symptom management
- Reduced masking pressure creates opportunities for authentic expression and energy conservation
- Life experience wisdom enables redefinition of success metrics around sustainability and personal meaning
- Late diagnosis or deeper self-understanding facilitates identity integration and authentic living
- Second act opportunities allow for meaningful contribution that leverages neurodivergent perspectives as strengths

Chapter 8: Medical Advocacy - Getting the Help You Need

Dr. Sarah Chen had been practicing family medicine for fifteen years when 48-year-old Patricia walked into her office with a three-page typed document. "Doctor," Patricia said, setting the papers on the exam table, "I need your help figuring out what's happening to me, and I've brought evidence."

Patricia's story would become a turning point in Dr. Chen's understanding of AuDHD in women. The document contained months of symptom tracking, research citations, and clear requests for specific tests. Patricia had done something many AuDHD women never learn to do—she had become her own medical advocate.

"I spent forty-eight years being dismissed by doctors who told me my symptoms were 'stress' or 'just part of being a woman,'" Patricia explained. "I'm not leaving here without answers this time."

Patricia's approach worked. Within six months, she had her AuDHD diagnosis, appropriate hormone testing, and a treatment plan that acknowledged both her neurological differences and her hormonal needs. Her success came from understanding a crucial truth: effective medical advocacy for AuDHD women requires preparation, persistence, and strategic communication.

Finding AuDHD-Informed Providers

The first challenge many AuDHD women face involves finding healthcare providers who understand both autism and ADHD, particularly how these conditions present in women across different life stages.

The Provider Knowledge Gap

Research from multiple sources reveals significant gaps in healthcare provider knowledge about AuDHD in women. Many doctors receive minimal training about autism and ADHD beyond childhood presentations, and even fewer understand how hormonal fluctuations affect neurodivergent symptoms.

Red Flags in Provider Responses:

- Dismissing symptoms as "normal stress" without investigation
- Focusing solely on mental health without considering neurological factors
- Unfamiliarity with female presentations of autism and ADHD
- Resistance to hormonal testing or treatment considerations
- Immediate prescription of antidepressants without comprehensive evaluation

Green Flags for AuDHD-Informed Care:

- Willingness to learn about conditions they're less familiar with
- Recognition that autism and ADHD can co-occur
- Understanding of hormonal influences on neurological symptoms
- Collaborative approach to diagnosis and treatment
- Respect for patient expertise about their own experiences

Case Example: The Education Partnership

Maria found her ideal provider through an unexpected partnership. Dr. Williams, a gynecologist, was honest about her limited AuDHD knowledge but willing to learn.

"She told me, 'I don't know much about autism and ADHD in women, but I'm willing to research and work with you to figure this out,'" Maria recalled. "That honesty and willingness to learn meant more to me than finding someone who claimed to be an expert but didn't really understand my experience."

Maria and Dr. Williams developed a collaborative relationship:

- Maria brought research articles about AuDHD and hormones

- Dr. Williams consulted with specialists and attended relevant training
- They developed treatment plans based on current research and Maria's tracked symptoms
- Regular follow-ups allowed for adjustments based on Maria's responses

Finding Providers Through Strategic Searching

Locating AuDHD-informed providers requires targeted strategies:

Specialist Networks: Look for providers who work with autism, ADHD, or women's hormonal health and ask about their experience with dual diagnoses.

Academic Medical Centers: University-affiliated providers often have more exposure to complex cases and current research.

Professional Organizations: Contact organizations like CHADD, the Autism Society, or women's health groups for provider recommendations.

Online Communities: Neurodivergent women's groups often share provider recommendations and experiences.

Referral Chains: Start with any supportive provider and ask for referrals to colleagues who might have more relevant expertise.

Case Example: The Referral Strategy

Jennifer used a strategic referral approach to build her healthcare team:

"I started with a therapist who understood autism in women. She referred me to a psychiatrist experienced with ADHD. The psychiatrist referred me to an endocrinologist who understood hormonal influences on brain function. Each provider learned from the others, and I ended up with a team that could coordinate my care."

Jennifer's team approach included:

- Primary care physician for general health monitoring
- Psychiatrist for ADHD medication management
- Endocrinologist for hormone evaluation and treatment
- Therapist for coping strategies and support
- Regular communication between providers about treatment coordination

Appointment Preparation Scripts and Templates

Effective medical advocacy requires structured preparation that presents information clearly and requests specific actions from providers.

The Pre-Appointment Preparation Framework

Successful appointments begin with thorough preparation that organizes information and clarifies goals:

Symptom Documentation: Detailed records of symptoms, patterns, and impacts on daily functioning.

Research Summary: Relevant studies or articles about AuDHD in women, particularly those related to current concerns.

Specific Requests: Clear list of desired tests, referrals, or treatments based on research and symptoms.

Question List: Prepared questions to ensure all concerns get addressed during the limited appointment time.

Case Example: The Documentation System

Linda developed a comprehensive documentation system for her appointments:

"I created a one-page summary for each appointment with four sections: current symptoms, pattern observations, research highlights, and specific requests. I also brought detailed symptom tracking data as backup. This kept me focused and helped doctors understand exactly what I needed."

Linda's one-page summary included:

- Current primary concerns with severity ratings
- Monthly patterns related to hormonal cycles
- Relevant research citations with key points highlighted
- Specific tests or referrals requested
- Questions requiring answers

Appointment Communication Scripts

Structured communication helps ensure important information gets conveyed effectively:

Opening Statement Script: "I'm here because I'm experiencing symptoms that research suggests may be related to AuDHD and hormonal fluctuations. I've been tracking my symptoms and have some specific questions and requests based on current research."

Symptom Presentation Script: "My main concerns are [specific symptoms] which follow a pattern of [frequency/timing]. These symptoms impact my [work/relationships/daily functioning] in the following ways: [specific examples]."

Research Presentation Script: "I've found research suggesting that [specific finding] might explain my symptoms. I've brought a summary of the key studies and would like to discuss how this might apply to my situation."

Request Script: "Based on my symptoms and the research I've found, I'd like to request [specific tests/referrals/treatments]. Could we discuss these options and determine what might be appropriate for my situation?"

Follow-Up Planning Script: "What are our next steps? When should I follow up? What should I monitor or track between now and our next appointment?"

Case Example: The Structured Approach

Rebecca used scripts to transform her appointment experiences:

"Before I started using scripts, I'd get flustered and forget half of what I wanted to say. With preparation, I could stay focused and make sure doctors understood what I needed. The scripts helped me sound confident and knowledgeable rather than scattered and emotional."

Rebecca's approach included:

- Writing out key points in advance
- Practicing delivery to reduce anxiety
- Bringing written copies to reference during appointments
- Taking notes during provider responses
- Confirming understanding before leaving

Hormone Testing Protocols and Interpretation

Understanding hormonal influences on AuDHD symptoms requires appropriate testing and informed interpretation of results.

Essential Hormone Tests for AuDHD Women

Comprehensive hormonal evaluation should include tests that assess reproductive hormones, stress hormones, and thyroid function:

Reproductive Hormones:

- Estradiol (estrogen) - multiple tests across the cycle
- Progesterone - tested during luteal phase
- Testosterone - free and total levels
- FSH and LH - to assess reproductive status

Stress and Adrenal Hormones:

- Cortisol - ideally measured multiple times daily
- DHEA-S - indicates adrenal function
- Pregnenolone - precursor hormone

Thyroid Function:

- TSH, Free T3, Free T4 - comprehensive thyroid panel
- Reverse T3 - indicates conversion issues
- Thyroid antibodies - to rule out autoimmune conditions

Case Example: The Comprehensive Testing

Amanda's hormone testing revealed patterns that explained her cyclical symptoms:

"My estradiol levels were swinging wildly - sometimes three times higher than normal, then crashing to menopausal levels within days. My cortisol was elevated all day, and my progesterone was almost undetectable. Finally, I had data that explained why I felt like different people on different days."

Amanda's results showed:

- Erratic estradiol fluctuations consistent with perimenopause
- Chronically elevated cortisol suggesting stress system dysfunction
- Low progesterone contributing to sleep and anxiety issues
- Normal thyroid function ruling out that as a contributing factor

Timing Considerations for Hormone Testing

For women with regular cycles, timing of hormone tests affects interpretation:

Day 3 Testing: Tests baseline hormone levels for FSH, LH, and estradiol during early follicular phase.

Day 21 Testing: Measures progesterone during presumed luteal phase to confirm ovulation.

Multiple Time Points: For women with irregular cycles or perimenopause, multiple tests across time provide better pattern recognition.

Salivary vs. Blood Testing: Salivary tests measure active hormone levels, while blood tests measure total levels including bound hormones.

Interpreting Results in AuDHD Context

Hormone test interpretation for AuDHD women requires understanding how neurological differences might affect optimal hormone ranges:

Individual Variation: AuDHD women may function better with hormone levels in different ranges than neurotypical women.

Symptom Correlation: Test results should be interpreted alongside symptom patterns rather than just reference ranges.

Medication Interactions: ADHD medications and other treatments may affect hormone levels and interpretation.

Cycle Pattern Analysis: For cycling women, patterns of change may be more informative than absolute values.

Case Example: The Context-Dependent Interpretation

Sarah's hormone levels were "normal" according to lab ranges but problematic for her AuDHD brain:

"My doctor said my estrogen levels were fine, but when I looked at the actual numbers alongside my symptom tracking, I could see that my ADHD symptoms were worst when my estrogen was in the lower part of the 'normal' range. For my brain, those levels weren't optimal."

Sarah's interpretation included:

- Correlation analysis between hormone levels and symptom severity
- Recognition that "normal" ranges are population averages, not individual optimization
- Adjustment of treatment goals to achieve symptom improvement rather than just "normal" numbers
- Ongoing monitoring to establish personal optimal ranges

Self-Advocacy When Doctors Dismiss Concerns

Unfortunately, many AuDHD women encounter dismissive attitudes from healthcare providers. Effective self-advocacy strategies can help overcome these barriers.

Common Dismissive Responses and Counter-Strategies

"This is just stress" Counter: "I understand stress can cause symptoms, but I've been tracking these patterns for months, and they correlate with my menstrual cycle rather than stress levels. I'd like to rule out hormonal causes before attributing everything to stress."

"You don't look autistic" Counter: "Research shows that autism presents differently in women and is often missed. I've brought information about female presentations and would like to discuss assessment options."

"ADHD is overdiagnosed these days" Counter: "Actually, research shows ADHD is underdiagnosed in women. I've documented specific symptoms and their impact on my functioning. Could we discuss evaluation options?"

"Have you tried just relaxing/exercising/eating better?" Counter: "I appreciate lifestyle factors are important, but these symptoms persist despite good self-care. I'd like to investigate potential medical causes alongside lifestyle approaches."

The Persistence Strategy

Effective advocacy sometimes requires persistent repetition of requests:

Document Everything: Keep records of all appointments, requests made, and responses received.

Repeat Requests: If reasonable requests are denied, ask for documentation of why they're being refused.

Second Opinions: When initial providers are unhelpful, seek evaluations from different doctors.

Escalation Paths: Understand complaint processes within healthcare systems when providers are unresponsive.

Case Example: The Documentation Defense

Kelly used documentation to advocate effectively for hormone testing:

"My first doctor dismissed my request for hormone testing, saying I was 'too young for menopause' at 42. I documented her refusal and sought a second opinion. The new doctor did the testing and found I was indeed in perimenopause. Having documentation of the first doctor's dismissal helped validate my advocacy with the second provider."

Kelly's documentation included:

- Written summaries of each appointment
- Copies of requests that were denied
- Symptom tracking data showing hormone-related patterns
- Research supporting her requests
- Clear timeline of advocacy efforts

Building Provider Relationships

Long-term advocacy benefits from developing collaborative relationships with healthcare providers:

Educational Partnership: Share relevant research and invite providers to learn alongside you.

Mutual Respect: Acknowledge provider expertise while asserting your own knowledge of your experiences.

Clear Communication: Use professional, specific language to describe symptoms and requests.

Reasonable Expectations: Understand that complex conditions may require time and multiple appointments to address fully.

Case Example: The Collaborative Success

Through patient advocacy, Jennifer transformed her relationship with her primary care doctor:

"Initially, Dr. Martinez was skeptical about my AuDHD concerns. But I kept bringing good research, tracking detailed symptoms, and asking reasonable questions. Over six months, she became genuinely interested in learning about neurodivergent women. Now she refers other patients to me for resources and has even attended training about ADHD in women."

Jennifer's collaborative approach included:

- Bringing high-quality research articles with key points highlighted
- Asking for her doctor's perspective on findings rather than demanding specific treatments
- Sharing resources that might help other patients
- Expressing appreciation for her doctor's willingness to learn
- Maintaining realistic timelines for complex evaluations

Building Your Medical Advocacy Skills

Effective medical advocacy develops over time through practice and experience:

Knowledge Building: Continuously learn about AuDHD, hormonal influences, and current research.

Communication Skills: Practice presenting information clearly and professionally.

Documentation Habits: Develop systems for tracking symptoms, appointments, and treatment responses.

Support Networks: Connect with other AuDHD women who can share advocacy strategies and provider recommendations.

Self-Care Integration: Recognize that advocacy can be exhausting and build in recovery time.

The journey toward effective medical advocacy transforms AuDHD women from passive patients into active partners in their healthcare. This shift requires courage, preparation, and persistence, but the rewards—appropriate diagnosis, effective treatment, and respectful provider relationships—make the effort worthwhile.

Patricia's three-page document that day represented more than symptom tracking—it represented a fundamental change in how she approached her healthcare. By becoming an informed advocate for her own needs, she opened the door to understanding and treatment that had eluded her for decades.

The Advocacy Transformation

Medical advocacy for AuDHD women isn't just about getting better healthcare—it's about reclaiming agency in medical relationships that have too often dismissed or minimized women's experiences. When AuDHD women become effective advocates, they not only improve their own care but also help educate providers who may better serve other neurodivergent women in the future.

The skills developed through medical advocacy extend beyond healthcare settings, building confidence and communication abilities that benefit all areas of life. AuDHD women who learn to advocate effectively in medical settings often find they can apply these skills to workplace accommodations, educational supports, and relationship communication.

Core Advocacy Principles for Medical Success

- Finding AuDHD-informed providers requires strategic searching and often involves educating willing providers about neurodivergent presentations
- Structured appointment preparation with documentation and scripts ensures important information gets communicated effectively
- Comprehensive hormone testing with appropriate timing and interpretation provides crucial data for understanding symptom patterns
- Persistent self-advocacy with professional communication helps overcome dismissive attitudes and builds collaborative provider relationships
- Developing advocacy skills transforms healthcare experiences from frustrating encounters to productive partnerships focused on optimal health outcomes

Chapter 9: Daily Life Hacks for Hormonal Fluctuations

The notification chimed on Lisa's phone at 6 AM: "Cycle Day 23 - Low Energy Predicted. Activate Survival Mode Protocol." This wasn't a medical alert or emergency warning—it was Lisa's personalized hormone tracking system reminding her that today would likely be challenging for her AuDHD brain.

By 8 AM, Lisa had already implemented her "survival mode" strategies: she'd laid out comfortable clothes the night before, prepared easy meals in advance, moved her most demanding work tasks to tomorrow, and set up her sensory regulation toolkit within arm's reach. What would have been a day of struggle and self-criticism had become a manageable experience guided by self-knowledge and preparation.

"Understanding my hormonal patterns changed everything," Lisa reflected. "Instead of being surprised by bad days and wondering what was wrong with me, I could predict and prepare. I stopped fighting my biology and started working with it."

Lisa's approach represents a fundamental shift in managing AuDHD symptoms—from reactive coping to proactive planning based on hormonal patterns and neurological needs.

Cycle-Synced Energy Management

The foundation of effective daily life management for AuDHD women lies in understanding and working with natural energy fluctuations rather than against them.

Understanding Your Energy Signature

Every AuDHD woman has a unique "energy signature"—patterns of cognitive capacity, emotional regulation, and physical energy that fluctuate predictably across hormonal cycles. Identifying these patterns enables strategic life planning.

High-Energy Characteristics:

- Enhanced focus and concentration abilities
- Improved medication effectiveness
- Better stress tolerance and emotional regulation
- Increased social capacity and communication skills
- Higher physical energy and motivation

Low-Energy Characteristics:

- Reduced attention span and increased distractibility
- Heightened sensory sensitivities
- Decreased emotional regulation and stress tolerance
- Social exhaustion and communication difficulties
- Physical fatigue and reduced motivation

Case Example: The Energy Mapping Project

Maria spent three months mapping her energy patterns and discovered a predictable cycle:

"Days 1-7: Recovery phase—gentle activities, basic self-care, minimal social demands. Days 8-14: Power phase—tackle big projects, schedule important meetings, handle challenging conversations. Days 15-18: Transition phase—moderate demands, begin preparing for low-energy period. Days 19-28: Survival phase— maintain essentials only, maximum self-care, avoid new stressors."

Maria's energy mapping included:

- Daily ratings of cognitive capacity on a 1-10 scale
- Medication effectiveness tracking
- Sensory sensitivity monitoring
- Social energy availability assessment
- Physical energy and motivation levels
- Sleep quality and requirements

Energy-Based Task Allocation

Once energy patterns are identified, tasks can be strategically allocated to optimize success and minimize struggle:

High-Energy Task Categories:

- Complex problem-solving and decision-making
- Important communications and difficult conversations
- Learning new skills or tackling challenging projects
- Social obligations and networking activities
- Major life decisions and planning

Low-Energy Task Categories:

- Routine maintenance and familiar activities
- Creative pursuits and relaxing hobbies
- Gentle exercise and restorative practices
- Organizing and decluttering spaces
- Self-care and recovery activities

Moderate-Energy Task Categories:

- Regular work responsibilities and routine tasks
- Light social activities with trusted people
- Household management and planning
- Health appointments and routine check-ups
- Moderate exercise and enjoyable activities

Case Example: The Strategic Calendar

Jennifer redesigned her entire scheduling approach around energy cycles:

"I stopped trying to maintain consistent productivity and started planning around my natural rhythms. I schedule presentations and important meetings during my high-energy weeks. I batch routine tasks during moderate-energy periods. I protect my low-energy time for recovery and gentle activities."

102

Jennifer's strategic calendar included:

- Color-coded scheduling based on predicted energy levels
- Flexible deadline management that accommodated cycle variations
- Buffer days around predictably difficult periods
- Backup plans for when energy predictions were incorrect
- Regular calendar reviews to adjust based on pattern changes

Energy Conservation Strategies

Effective energy management involves not just allocation but also conservation techniques that preserve capacity for essential activities:

Decision Fatigue Reduction: Minimize daily decisions through routines, meal planning, and wardrobe simplification.

Task Batching: Group similar activities together to reduce cognitive switching costs.

Transition Buffers: Build extra time between activities to accommodate processing differences.

Energy Recovery: Schedule specific recovery time after demanding activities.

Sensory Regulation Toolkits for Difficult Days

AuDHD women experience heightened sensory sensitivities during certain hormonal phases, making comprehensive sensory regulation tools essential for daily functioning.

Building Your Sensory Toolkit

Effective sensory regulation requires tools that address multiple sensory systems and can be easily accessed during difficult periods:

Auditory Regulation Tools:

- Noise-canceling headphones for overwhelming environments
- White noise or nature sounds for focus and calming
- Specific music playlists for different regulation needs
- Earplugs for situations where headphones aren't appropriate

Visual Regulation Tools:

- Sunglasses for light sensitivity management
- Blue light filtering glasses for screen time
- Soft lighting options for home and work environments
- Visual comfort items like calming pictures or colors

Tactile Regulation Tools:

- Weighted blankets for deep pressure input
- Fidget toys and tactile objects for self-regulation
- Soft textures for comfort during distress
- Compression clothing for proprioceptive input

Olfactory Regulation Tools:

- Essential oils for calming or alerting as needed
- Unscented personal care products to avoid overwhelm
- Scent-neutralizing options for sensitivity management
- Pleasant scents for mood regulation and comfort

Case Example: The Mobile Sensory Kit

Rachel assembled what she called her "survival kit" for difficult sensory days:

"I keep a small bag with essentials: noise-canceling earbuds, sunglasses, peppermint oil, a soft scarf, and fidget cube. Having these tools accessible means I can handle unexpected sensory challenges without falling apart. The kit has saved me from countless meltdowns."

Rachel's mobile kit included:

- Compact noise-canceling earbuds for discrete use
- Lightweight sunglasses that fit in any bag
- Small container of calming essential oil
- Soft, comforting fabric piece for tactile needs
- Discrete fidget tool for focus and regulation

Sensory Environment Modification

Beyond personal tools, creating supportive sensory environments at home and work enhances daily functioning:

Home Environment Modifications:

- Lighting controls to adjust brightness and color temperature
- Sound management through carpets, curtains, and wall treatments
- Temperature control for comfort and regulation
- Organized spaces that reduce visual overwhelm
- Designated quiet areas for sensory recovery

Workplace Environment Modifications:

- Desk positioning to minimize distracting stimuli
- Personal lighting and sound management tools
- Organization systems that reduce visual clutter
- Access to quiet spaces for sensory breaks
- Communication with colleagues about sensory needs

Case Example: The Sanctuary Spaces

Linda created what she called "sanctuary spaces" in both her home and office:

"I have a corner of my bedroom with soft lighting, comfortable textures, and calming colors where I go when I'm overwhelmed. At work, I negotiated for a desk in a quieter area and permission to use noise-canceling headphones. These spaces give me places to regulate when my sensory system is overloaded."

Linda's sanctuary spaces included:

- Consistent sensory elements across environments
- Easy access during difficult periods
- Tools for quick sensory regulation
- Visual cues that promoted calmness
- Minimal stimuli to allow nervous system recovery

Sensory Regulation Techniques

Effective sensory regulation involves both tools and techniques that can be implemented quickly during challenging moments:

Deep Pressure Techniques: Self-hugs, weighted items, or gentle compression to calm overactive nervous systems.

Breathing Regulation: Structured breathing patterns that activate parasympathetic nervous system responses.

Movement Integration: Gentle movement or exercise to help process sensory input and regulate energy.

Mindful Awareness: Techniques for identifying sensory overwhelm before it becomes unmanageable.

Executive Function Supports That Work

Hormonal fluctuations significantly impact executive function abilities in AuDHD women, requiring flexible support systems that adapt to changing cognitive capacity.

Core Executive Function Challenges

AuDHD women experience executive function difficulties that worsen during certain hormonal phases:

Task Initiation Problems: Difficulty starting activities, especially during low-motivation periods.

Working Memory Issues: Challenges holding information in mind while completing complex tasks.

Cognitive Flexibility Deficits: Difficulty switching between tasks or adapting to unexpected changes.

Planning and Organization Struggles: Problems with sequential thinking and long-term planning.

Time Management Difficulties: Challenges with time estimation, prioritization, and deadline management.

The External Brain System

Effective executive function support often involves creating "external brain" systems that supplement internal cognitive abilities:

Digital External Brain Tools:

- Task management apps that break projects into manageable steps
- Calendar systems with multiple reminders and alerts
- Note-taking apps that capture and organize information
- Habit tracking tools that support routine development
- Timer and focus apps that support attention management

Physical External Brain Tools:

- Visual planning boards and charts
- Color-coded organization systems
- Physical reminder systems and cues
- Structured filing and storage systems
- Written checklists and procedures

Case Example: The Hybrid System

Susan developed what she called her "hybrid external brain" combining digital and physical tools:

"I use my phone for reminders and scheduling, but I need physical visual cues too. I have a whiteboard calendar, color-coded files, and visual checklists. The combination helps me stay organized even when my internal executive function is struggling."

Susan's hybrid system included:

- Digital calendar with multiple alarm types and notifications
- Physical whiteboard for visual planning and daily priorities
- Color-coded filing system for important documents
- Written procedures for routine tasks and processes
- Visual progress tracking for long-term projects

Flexible Planning Strategies

Executive function support must accommodate the fluctuating nature of AuDHD symptoms:

Good Day/Bad Day Planning: Different organizational approaches for different cognitive capacity levels.

Multiple Backup Systems: Redundant systems that ensure important tasks don't get forgotten.

Energy-Matched Task Difficulty: Pairing task complexity with available cognitive resources.

Recovery Period Integration: Building in time for cognitive rest and restoration.

Case Example: The Three-Tier System

Angela developed a three-tier planning system that adapted to her cognitive capacity:

"Tier 1 is for high-function days—complex projects, important decisions, challenging tasks. Tier 2 is for moderate days—routine work, maintenance tasks, familiar activities. Tier 3 is for survival days—essentials only, gentle activities, maximum support systems."

Angela's three-tier system included:

- Pre-planned task lists for each capacity level
- Flexible deadlines that accommodated cognitive fluctuations
- Support tool accessibility at every tier
- Clear criteria for determining daily tier assignment
- Regular system evaluation and adjustment

Communication Strategies for Hormonal Phases

Hormonal fluctuations affect communication abilities, requiring adaptive strategies that accommodate changing social and linguistic capacity.

Communication Capacity Fluctuations

AuDHD women experience predictable changes in communication abilities across hormonal cycles:

High-Capacity Communication Characteristics:

- Enhanced verbal fluency and articulation
- Better social reading and interpretation abilities
- Improved conflict resolution and negotiation skills
- Increased tolerance for complex conversations
- Better emotional regulation during interactions

Low-Capacity Communication Characteristics:

- Reduced verbal fluency and word-finding difficulties
- Decreased social interpretation abilities
- Heightened sensitivity to criticism or conflict
- Reduced tolerance for complex or lengthy conversations
- Increased likelihood of misunderstandings

Adaptive Communication Strategies

Understanding communication fluctuations enables strategic adaptation of interaction approaches:

High-Capacity Period Strategies:

- Schedule important conversations and negotiations
- Address complex relationship issues
- Engage in challenging professional communications
- Participate in social activities and networking events
- Handle conflict resolution and difficult discussions

Low-Capacity Period Strategies:

- Use written communication when possible
- Request extra processing time for important decisions
- Limit social obligations and complex interactions
- Use communication scripts for routine interactions
- Postpone non-urgent difficult conversations

Case Example: The Communication Calendar

Michelle integrated communication planning into her cycle tracking:

"I learned to schedule important conversations during my high-communication weeks and protect my low-communication periods. I let my family and close colleagues know about my patterns so they understand when I need extra patience or prefer written communication."

Michelle's communication calendar included:

- Monthly planning of important conversations based on predicted capacity
- Communication preference alerts for family and trusted colleagues
- Written communication templates for difficult periods
- Recovery time built in after challenging interactions

- Flexible rescheduling options for unexpected low-capacity days

Relationship Communication Strategies

Hormonal communication fluctuations require specific strategies for maintaining healthy relationships:

Partner Communication:

- Education about hormonal impacts on communication
- Clear signals about current communication capacity
- Written communication options during difficult periods
- Patience and understanding agreements during low-capacity times
- Appreciation expression during high-capacity periods

Workplace Communication:

- Professional language for explaining communication needs
- Email preferences during low-capacity periods
- Meeting scheduling around predicted communication abilities
- Clear documentation of important communications
- Colleague education about communication differences

Case Example: The Signal System

David and his AuDHD partner Sarah developed a communication signal system:

"Sarah uses a simple color system to let me know her communication capacity—green means normal interaction, yellow means be patient and keep it simple, red means minimal talking and written communication preferred. It helps me adjust my expectations and communication style to match her current abilities."

Their signal system included:

- Simple visual cues that could be easily updated
- Clear behavioral guidelines for each communication level
- Written alternatives for important conversations during red periods
- Appreciation rituals for successful navigation of difficult periods
- Regular system evaluation and adjustment based on effectiveness

Professional Communication Adaptations

Workplace communication requires professional strategies that accommodate hormonal fluctuations without revealing personal information:

Email Management: Using email for complex communications during low-capacity periods to allow processing time.

Meeting Preparation: Extra preparation during low-capacity periods to compensate for reduced verbal fluency.

Boundary Setting: Professional ways to request communication accommodations without disclosing personal details.

Colleague Education: General information about communication differences that doesn't require personal disclosure.

Daily life management for AuDHD women becomes dramatically more effective when hormonal patterns are understood and accommodated rather than fought against. The strategies that work—cycle-synced energy management, comprehensive sensory regulation, flexible executive function supports, and adaptive communication approaches—all share a common theme: working with neurological differences rather than against them.

Lisa's morning notification system represents more than just good planning—it represents a fundamental shift from self-criticism to self-compassion, from struggling against biology to partnering with it. When AuDHD women develop these daily life hacks, they transform from victims of unpredictable symptoms to architects of sustainable, authentic lives.

The Integration Journey

The journey toward effective daily life management requires patience, experimentation, and self-compassion. AuDHD women often need time to identify their unique patterns, develop effective tools, and integrate new strategies into existing routines. The goal isn't perfection but rather sustainable approaches that honor both neurological differences and hormonal fluctuations.

As women develop expertise in managing their daily AuDHD experience, they often find that these skills transfer to other areas of life, including workplace success and career satisfaction. The self-knowledge and adaptive strategies that make daily life manageable also contribute to professional effectiveness and authentic career development.

Essential Daily Management Elements

- Cycle-synced energy management optimizes productivity by aligning tasks with natural capacity fluctuations
- Comprehensive sensory regulation toolkits provide immediate access to regulation strategies during challenging periods
- Flexible executive function supports adapt to changing cognitive capacity while maintaining essential functioning
- Adaptive communication strategies accommodate hormonal influences on social and linguistic abilities
- Self-compassionate planning approaches honor biological realities rather than fighting against natural patterns

Chapter 10: Workplace Strategies Across Life Stages

The email arrived at 3:47 PM on a Friday: "Due to budget constraints, we're implementing an open office plan. All personal offices will be converted to collaborative workspace. The transition begins Monday." For 52-year-old marketing director Carmen, this wasn't just an inconvenience—it was a crisis that threatened the carefully constructed accommodations that had allowed her to thrive professionally for the past decade.

Carmen's corner office wasn't a luxury—it was a necessity. The quiet space, controlled lighting, and freedom from sudden interruptions had been the foundation of her professional success since her AuDHD diagnosis at 45. Now, facing perimenopause symptoms that had already intensified her sensory sensitivities, the prospect of an open office felt insurmountable.

"I had two choices," Carmen recalled. "I could accept defeat and start looking for early retirement options, or I could advocate for what I needed to continue contributing meaningfully. I chose to fight."

Carmen's story illustrates a crucial reality: workplace success for AuDHD women requires ongoing adaptation, strategic accommodation, and skilled advocacy that evolves across life stages and career phases.

Hormonal Accommodation Negotiations

One of the most challenging aspects of workplace advocacy for AuDHD women involves communicating the need for accommodations that fluctuate with hormonal changes—a concept that many employers struggle to understand.

The Challenge of Fluctuating Needs

Traditional workplace accommodations assume consistent, predictable needs. But AuDHD women experience accommodation requirements that change based on hormonal cycles, life stages, and stress levels, creating unique advocacy challenges.

Static vs. Dynamic Accommodation Needs:

- Static needs remain consistent (noise-canceling headphones, written instructions)
- Dynamic needs fluctuate predictably (flexible deadlines during difficult cycle phases)
- Crisis accommodations address temporary but severe challenges (perimenopause symptom management)
- Preventive accommodations reduce the likelihood of accommodation crises

Case Example: The Cycle-Aware Schedule

Maria, a project manager, successfully negotiated what she called "cycle-aware scheduling":

"I explained to my supervisor that my productivity and cognitive capacity follow predictable monthly patterns. I proposed scheduling demanding presentations and deadlines during my high-functioning weeks while protecting my low-energy periods for routine tasks and recovery. The result was better work quality and more consistent performance."

Maria's accommodation package included:

- Flexible deadline management based on monthly capacity cycles
- Project scheduling that aligned complex work with high-energy periods
- Written documentation of all important communications
- Permission to work from home during sensory-challenging periods
- Regular check-ins to assess accommodation effectiveness

Language Strategies for Hormonal Accommodations

Effective accommodation requests require professional language that explains needs without oversharing personal information:

Professional Framing: "I experience predictable cycles in my cognitive capacity and would benefit from flexible scheduling to optimize my productivity."

Research-Based Rationale: "Research shows that many women experience monthly fluctuations in executive function and attention, and accommodating these patterns can improve overall performance."

Benefit-Focused Communication: "This accommodation would allow me to consistently deliver high-quality work while managing natural variations in my cognitive resources."

Collaborative Approach: "I'd like to work together to develop a system that ensures my best work while accommodating my neurological differences."

Case Example: The Strategic Disclosure

Jennifer developed a strategic approach to accommodation requests that balanced disclosure with professional presentation:

"I focused on my work needs rather than my diagnosis. I explained that I have neurological differences that affect my attention and sensory processing, and that research-backed accommodations would help me perform at my best. I brought examples of how similar accommodations had worked in other organizations."

Jennifer's strategy included:

- Focus on work performance rather than personal struggles
- Research citations supporting requested accommodations
- Examples from other organizations implementing similar strategies
- Clear metrics for measuring accommodation success

- Regular evaluation and adjustment processes

Documenting Accommodation Effectiveness

Successful accommodation negotiations often require evidence of effectiveness:

Performance Metrics: Document improvements in work quality, productivity, and job satisfaction with accommodations.

Comparative Analysis: Show performance differences with and without accommodations to demonstrate their value.

Colleague Impact: Document how accommodations improve not just individual performance but team dynamics and outcomes.

Cost-Benefit Analysis: Demonstrate that accommodation costs are minimal compared to the benefits of retaining skilled employees.

Career Navigation During Perimenopause

Perimenopause presents unique workplace challenges for AuDHD women as hormonal chaos intersects with peak career responsibilities and aging workplace dynamics.

The Perimenopause Career Crisis

Many AuDHD women experience career crises during perimenopause as previously effective coping strategies become inadequate for managing intensified symptoms:

Cognitive Challenges: Brain fog, memory issues, and attention difficulties that affect job performance.

Sensory Intensification: Increased sensitivity to workplace stimuli like noise, lighting, and interruptions.

Energy Fluctuations: Unpredictable energy patterns that make consistent performance challenging.

Emotional Regulation: Difficulty managing workplace stress and interpersonal challenges.

Case Example: The Executive's Adaptation

Susan, a 48-year-old VP of Operations, faced a perimenopause-driven career crisis:

"I'd built my reputation on being the person who could handle anything, anytime. Suddenly, I couldn't concentrate in meetings, office noise made me anxious, and I needed recovery time after every challenging interaction. I felt like I was failing at everything I'd previously mastered."

Susan's perimenopause impact included:

- Difficulty processing information during fast-paced meetings
- Sensory overload from open office environments
- Energy crashes that affected afternoon productivity
- Increased difficulty with task switching and interruptions
- Anxiety about performance decline and job security

Strategic Career Adaptations

Successful perimenopause career navigation requires strategic adaptations that leverage strengths while accommodating new limitations:

Role Modification: Adjusting job responsibilities to align with changing capacities and strengths.

Schedule Optimization: Restructuring work schedules around energy patterns and symptom fluctuations.

Environment Control: Creating or negotiating for work environments that support cognitive function.

Support System Development: Building workplace relationships that provide understanding and assistance.

Skill Leveraging: Emphasizing accumulated expertise and institutional knowledge while managing newer challenges.

Case Example: The Consultant's Transformation

Patricia transformed her career approach during perimenopause:

"Instead of fighting my changing brain, I redesigned my work around it. I moved from high-stress client management to strategic consulting where I could leverage my deep expertise. I negotiated for project-based work that allowed me to manage my energy and focus on what I do best."

Patricia's transformation included:

- Shift from management to individual contributor role emphasizing expertise
- Project-based work structure that accommodated energy fluctuations
- Remote work arrangements that controlled sensory environment
- Flexible scheduling that aligned with optimal performance times
- Mentoring responsibilities that utilized accumulated wisdom

Workplace Advocacy During Perimenopause

Perimenopause advocacy requires balancing disclosure decisions with accommodation needs:

Medical Documentation: Working with healthcare providers to document perimenopause symptoms and their workplace impact.

Accommodation Planning: Developing comprehensive accommodation requests that address multiple symptoms.

Performance Protection: Creating documentation trails that protect against performance-based discrimination.

Resource Identification: Connecting with EAP services, HR resources, and legal protections.

Case Example: The Proactive Approach

Linda took a proactive approach to perimenopause workplace advocacy:

"I knew perimenopause was coming and prepared for it professionally. I researched my legal rights, documented my accommodation needs, and had conversations with HR before my symptoms became crisis-level. This preparation allowed me to navigate the transition while maintaining my career trajectory."

Linda's proactive strategy included:

- Educational sessions with HR about perimenopause and workplace impact
- Development of flexible accommodation plans before crisis periods
- Documentation of successful accommodation strategies
- Building support networks with other women facing similar challenges
- Legal consultation about rights and protections

Entrepreneurship Advantages for AuDHD Women

Many AuDHD women find entrepreneurship provides unique advantages that align with their neurological differences and accommodation needs.

Why Entrepreneurship Appeals to AuDHD Women

Self-employment addresses many workplace challenges that AuDHD women face in traditional employment:

Environmental Control: Complete control over work environment, including sensory factors.

Schedule Flexibility: Ability to structure work around energy patterns and hormonal cycles.

Task Selection: Focus on strengths and interests while minimizing challenging areas.

Accommodation Freedom: No need to negotiate accommodations or explain neurological differences.

Authentic Expression: Freedom to work in ways that feel natural rather than forcing neurotypical performance.

Case Example: The Accidental Entrepreneur

Rebecca's entrepreneurship journey began from workplace accommodation failures:

"I kept getting fired from jobs where I was technically competent but couldn't handle the social and sensory demands. Finally, I started freelancing as a data analyst, working from home with clients who just wanted quality results. What began as desperation became the perfect career fit."

Rebecca's entrepreneurial advantages included:

- Complete sensory environment control working from home
- Project-based work that accommodated hyperfocus patterns
- Client relationships focused on deliverables rather than social performance
- Schedule flexibility that aligned with energy cycles
- Opportunity to specialize in areas of genuine interest and strength

Entrepreneurship Challenges for AuDHD Women

While entrepreneurship offers advantages, it also presents unique challenges that AuDHD women must navigate:

Executive Function Demands: Self-employment requires strong organizational and planning skills.

Networking Requirements: Business development often involves social interaction and relationship building.

Financial Management: Irregular income and complex financial planning can be challenging.

Client Communication: Professional communication and customer service demands.

Isolation Risks: Working alone can lead to social isolation and lack of support.

Strategic Entrepreneurship Approaches

Successful AuDHD entrepreneurs develop strategies that leverage their strengths while managing challenges:

Niche Specialization: Focusing on areas of genuine expertise and interest where AuDHD traits become advantages.

System Development: Creating robust systems and processes that support executive function challenges.

Support Team Building: Assembling teams or contractors to handle challenging areas like marketing or administration.

Client Education: Choosing and educating clients about working styles and communication preferences.

Work-Life Integration: Designing business models that support rather than conflict with personal needs.

Case Example: The Strategic Builder

Michelle built her consulting business around her AuDHD strengths:

"I realized that my attention to detail, pattern recognition, and systematic thinking were exactly what small businesses needed for process improvement. I built my practice around project-based consulting where I could hyperfocus on complex problems, deliver exceptional results, and then have recovery time before the next project."

Michelle's strategic approach included:

- Business model designed around hyperfocus abilities
- Client screening to find those who valued quality over speed
- Systematic approach to project management that utilized organizational strengths
- Partnership with other consultants to handle areas outside her expertise
- Marketing strategy that emphasized her unique analytical perspective

Building Sustainable Business Models

AuDHD entrepreneurs benefit from business models that accommodate their neurological differences:

Energy-Based Pricing: Pricing models that account for the quality and intensity of work rather than just time.

Flexible Scheduling: Business structures that allow for energy cycle management and recovery time.

Strength-Focused Services: Offerings that utilize AuDHD advantages like attention to detail, systematic thinking, and creative problem-solving.

Minimal Networking Models: Business development strategies that minimize traditional networking demands.

Technology Leverage: Using technology to handle routine tasks and communication challenges.

Neurodivergent Retirement Planning

Traditional retirement planning often assumes linear career progression and conventional life patterns—assumptions that may not apply to AuDHD women's career experiences.

Unique Retirement Considerations for AuDHD Women

AuDHD women face several retirement planning challenges that differ from neurotypical experiences:

Non-Linear Career Paths: Frequent job changes, career gaps, and late-career diagnoses can affect retirement savings.

Healthcare Cost Considerations: Ongoing medical needs and potential accommodation requirements.

Social Security Complications: Irregular work histories may affect benefit calculations.

Extended Working Years: Many AuDHD women find their stride later in life and may want or need to work longer.

Legacy and Meaning: Desire to contribute knowledge and experience to benefit other neurodivergent individuals.

Case Example: The Late-Career Flourishing

At 58, Diana was hitting her professional stride just as her peers were considering retirement:

"I didn't find work that truly fit until my fifties. My AuDHD traits became advantages in consulting rather than obstacles to overcome. I'm not ready to retire—I'm finally doing work that energizes rather than drains me. My retirement planning has to account for potentially working into my seventies by choice."

Diana's unique considerations included:

- Career peak occurring in traditional pre-retirement years
- Desire to continue meaningful work that utilized her strengths
- Need for flexible retirement that allowed continued contribution
- Healthcare planning that accommodated ongoing neurodivergent needs
- Legacy planning focused on mentoring other neurodivergent women

Alternative Retirement Models

AuDHD women often benefit from non-traditional retirement approaches:

Gradual Transition: Slowly reducing work responsibilities rather than abrupt retirement.

Portfolio Retirement: Combining part-time work, consulting, and personal projects.

Passion Pursuit: Focusing retirement years on previously deferred interests and special passions.

Mentorship Integration: Including formal or informal mentoring of neurodivergent individuals.

Advocacy Involvement: Participating in neurodiversity advocacy and education efforts.

Financial Planning Adaptations

Retirement financial planning for AuDHD women requires strategies that accommodate non-traditional career patterns:

Multiple Income Streams: Diversifying retirement income to accommodate potential continued work.

Healthcare Reserve Planning: Additional savings for ongoing medical and accommodation needs.

Flexibility Preservation: Maintaining options for changing life circumstances and interests.

Support System Integration: Planning for potential need for additional support services.

Case Example: The Comprehensive Planner

Margaret worked with a financial planner to develop a neurodivergent-informed retirement strategy:

"Traditional retirement planning assumed I'd want to stop working completely at 65. But my planner helped me create a flexible plan that accommodates my desire to continue meaningful work while ensuring I have security if my health or interests change. We planned for multiple scenarios rather than one fixed outcome."

Margaret's plan included:

- Flexible withdrawal strategies that accommodated continued earnings
- Healthcare savings accounts for ongoing neurodivergent-related expenses
- Investment in accessible housing and transportation
- Estate planning that included neurodiversity advocacy organizations
- Professional development funds for potential late-career pivots

Creating Meaning in Later Years

Many AuDHD women find their later years focused on meaning-making and contribution rather than traditional leisure retirement:

Knowledge Transfer: Sharing accumulated expertise with younger neurodivergent individuals.

Advocacy Work: Contributing to improved understanding and support for neurodivergent women.

Creative Pursuits: Finally having time and energy for long-deferred creative interests.

Community Building: Creating or supporting communities for neurodivergent individuals.

Research Participation: Contributing to research about neurodivergent experiences across the lifespan.

Carmen's open office crisis resolution became a model for other employees facing similar challenges. By advocating for a hybrid workspace solution—retaining some private spaces while creating collaborative areas—she not only solved her own accommodation needs but improved the workplace for many colleagues. Her success demonstrated that AuDHD workplace advocacy often benefits entire organizations.

The strategies that work across AuDHD women's career lifespans share common elements: self-knowledge, strategic advocacy, flexibility, and the courage to design work lives that honor both strengths and challenges. Whether navigating traditional employment, building entrepreneurial ventures, or planning for meaningful later years, success comes from working with rather than against neurological differences.

The Evolution of Workplace Success

Workplace success for AuDHD women isn't about overcoming their differences—it's about creating work environments and career paths that allow their unique strengths to flourish while providing necessary supports for areas of challenge. This evolution from accommodation to optimization represents a fundamental shift in how we think about neurodiversity in professional settings.

As more AuDHD women develop effective workplace strategies and advocacy skills, they create pathways for future generations while demonstrating that neurodivergent perspectives aren't just valuable—they're essential for innovative, inclusive, and successful organizations.

Professional Success Strategies Across Life Stages

- Hormonal accommodation negotiations require professional communication that focuses on work benefits rather than personal struggles
- Perimenopause career navigation demands strategic adaptations that leverage accumulated expertise while managing new challenges
- Entrepreneurship offers unique advantages for AuDHD women who can control their work environment and leverage their distinctive strengths
- Neurodivergent retirement planning accommodates non-linear career paths and the desire for continued meaningful contribution
- Successful workplace advocacy creates benefits not just for individual AuDHD women but for entire organizations seeking innovation and inclusion

Chapter 11: Building Your AuDHD Women's Support Network

The isolation that comes with being an AuDHD woman can feel suffocating. You've spent years wondering why you don't fit in, why social interactions drain you, why your mind works differently than everyone else's. The relief of understanding your neurodivergence often comes with a new challenge - finding your people. Building a support network isn't just about having friends; it's about creating a safety net of understanding, acceptance, and practical help that recognizes your unique needs as someone with both autism and ADHD.

Your support network becomes the foundation for everything else - your self-advocacy, your growth, your ability to thrive rather than merely survive. Without it, you're navigating a neurotypical world with a map written in a language you don't fully understand. With it, you have guides, translators, and fellow travelers who know the terrain.

Finding Community Online and Locally

Online Communities as Your Starting Point

The internet has revolutionized how neurodivergent women find each other. Facebook groups, Reddit communities, Discord servers, and specialized platforms like Mighty Networks host thousands of AuDHD women sharing experiences, strategies, and support. These digital spaces often become the first place you'll encounter others who truly understand your experience.

Sarah, a 34-year-old software developer, discovered an online AuDHD women's group after her diagnosis. "I posted about struggling with rejection sensitive dysphoria after a work meeting, and within hours I had fifteen responses from women who'd experienced the exact same thing. They shared coping strategies I'd never heard of and validation I'd never received. For the first time, I felt normal."

Look for groups that maintain clear community guidelines and active moderation. Red flags include groups that discourage seeking professional help, promote unproven treatments, or allow harmful content to persist. Quality online communities typically have pinned posts with resources, regular check-ins, and subgroups for specific topics like work, relationships, or parenting.

Local Community Building

While online connections provide immediate access to understanding, local communities offer face-to-face interaction and practical support. Start by checking with local autism organizations, libraries, community centers, and universities. Many areas have neurodiversity meetups, though they may not be specifically for AuDHD individuals.

Maria, a 28-year-old teacher, couldn't find an AuDHD group in her mid-sized city. She started by attending a general autism support group, where she met three other women who also had ADHD. They began meeting monthly at a quiet coffee shop, and within six months, their group had grown to twelve members through word-of-mouth and social media promotion.

Consider unconventional spaces too. Board game cafes, hobby groups, book clubs, and volunteer organizations often attract neurodivergent individuals. The key is finding activities that align with your interests and sensory needs while providing opportunities for genuine connection.

Navigating Online Platform Challenges

Each platform has its own culture and communication style. Facebook groups tend to be more conversational and personal, while Reddit communities often focus on information sharing and advice. Discord servers provide real-time chat but can be overwhelming for those with auditory processing differences.

Practice setting digital boundaries early. Turn off notifications during your focused work time, set specific hours for checking messages, and don't feel obligated to respond to every post or comment. Your online community should support your well-being, not create additional stress.

Starting or Joining Support Groups

Joining Existing Groups

Before joining any support group, research its format, leadership, and member demographics. Some groups are peer-led and informal, while others follow structured curricula with professional facilitators. Consider your communication preferences - do you prefer smaller, intimate settings or larger groups with diverse perspectives?

When you first attend, expect to feel anxious. This is normal and temporary. Most established groups have welcoming protocols for new members. Don't pressure yourself to share immediately; listening and observing helps you understand the group's dynamics and decide if it's a good fit.

Jennifer, a 41-year-old marketing manager, attended four different support groups before finding her community. "The first was too large and chaotic for my sensory sensitivities. The second focused only on challenges, which left me feeling worse. The third was perfect in size and balance, but met during my daughter's soccer practice. The fourth group met virtually in the evenings and had a wonderful mix of celebration and problem-solving. Persistence paid off."

Creating Your Own Group

If existing options don't meet your needs, consider starting your own group. This requires more energy and organization but allows you to create exactly what you need. Start small with three to five people and grow gradually.

Decide on your group's focus early. Will you concentrate on practical strategies, emotional support, social connection, or advocacy? Will you welcome family members or keep it AuDHD women only? These decisions shape everything from meeting format to ground rules.

Establish clear guidelines from the beginning. Address confidentiality, communication styles, conflict resolution, and group size limits. Many successful groups rotate facilitation responsibilities to prevent burnout and ensure diverse perspectives guide discussions.

Group Leadership Considerations

Leading a support group while managing your own AuDHD traits requires careful planning. Use your executive function strengths - many AuDHD women excel at organization and structure when they're interested in the topic. Create templates for meetings, maintain member contact lists, and develop systems for scheduling and communication.

Plan for your own needs too. Schedule recovery time after meetings, delegate tasks that drain you, and have backup plans for days when your symptoms are severe. The group should support you as much as you support it.

Partner and Family Education Approaches

Educating Romantic Partners

Your romantic partner's understanding directly impacts your daily stress levels and long-term relationship satisfaction. However, education must be approached strategically to avoid overwhelming them or triggering defensive responses.

Start with your most pressing needs rather than comprehensive autism and ADHD education. If sensory overload is your biggest challenge, begin there. Share specific examples of how your partner can help - dimming lights during conversations, using written communication for complex topics, or providing processing time before expecting responses.

Rachel, a 32-year-old graphic designer, used a gradual approach with her husband Mark. "I started by explaining why I needed our bedroom completely dark and quiet for sleep. Once he saw how much better I functioned with good sleep, he was more open to learning about other accommodations. We worked through one area at a time over several months."

Provide concrete resources rather than expecting your partner to research independently. Share specific articles, videos, or book chapters that resonate with your experience. Avoid overwhelming them with too much information at once.

Address common misconceptions directly but gently. Many partners struggle with invisible disability concepts or assume that strategies that work for neurotypical people will work for you. Explain that your needs aren't preferences or choices - they're neurological requirements for functioning.

Family System Changes

Educating family members requires different approaches depending on relationships and family dynamics. Parents may struggle with guilt about missed signs during childhood. Siblings might feel confused about changed family dynamics. Adult children may worry about their own traits.

Focus on practical changes that benefit the whole family. If family gatherings overwhelm your sensory system, suggest modifications that might help everyone - quieter music, smaller groups, or alternative activities. Frame accommodations as family improvements rather than special requirements for you.

Create family communication protocols that work with your processing style. Some families implement "24-hour rule" for important discussions, giving you time to process before responding.

Others use written communication for complex topics or family scheduling.

Workplace Education Strategies

Workplace education serves dual purposes - securing necessary accommodations and building understanding among colleagues. However, disclosure decisions are deeply personal and should be made carefully.

If you choose to disclose, focus on job performance and specific accommodations rather than diagnostic details. Explain how certain changes help you do your best work. For example, "I'm more productive with written project instructions rather than verbal ones" or "I work most effectively with consistent schedules and advance notice of changes."

Prepare for various responses. Some colleagues and supervisors will be immediately supportive, others may need time to understand, and a few might be resistant. Document accommodation requests and any resistance you encounter.

Consider partial disclosure for specific situations. You might explain sensory sensitivities without mentioning autism or discuss attention challenges without specifying ADHD. Gauge responses and adjust your approach accordingly.

Assembling Professional Support Teams

Core Team Members

Your professional support team should include medical providers who understand neurodivergence in women, mental health professionals trained in autism and ADHD, and specialists who address your specific challenges.

Primary care physicians anchor your medical team but may need education about AuDHD presentations in women. Prepare for appointments by bringing research about female autism and ADHD presentations, your specific symptoms, and questions about how your neurodivergence might affect other health concerns.

Mental health professionals should have specific training in both autism and ADHD, particularly in adult women. Cognitive-behavioral therapy, dialectical behavior therapy, and acceptance and commitment therapy have shown effectiveness for neurodivergent individuals when adapted appropriately.

Consider occupational therapists who specialize in sensory processing and executive function. They can assess your sensory profile, recommend environmental modifications, and teach strategies for daily living tasks.

Specialty Providers

Depending on your specific challenges, you might need additional specialists. Sleep medicine doctors can address common sleep issues in AuDHD individuals. Gastroenterologists understand the gut-brain connection that affects many neurodivergent people. Audiologists can assess auditory processing differences.

Nutritionists familiar with autism and ADHD can help address feeding difficulties, sensory food issues, or medication interactions with diet. Physical therapists who understand proprioceptive and vestibular differences can help with coordination and body awareness challenges.

Building Provider Relationships

Good provider relationships require active participation from you. Prepare for appointments with written lists of concerns, questions, and examples. Many AuDHD women struggle with medical advocacy in the moment, so preparation is essential.

Keep detailed records of symptoms, medication effects, and strategy effectiveness. Many providers appreciate patients who track their experiences systematically. Use apps, journals, or spreadsheets - whatever system you'll actually maintain.

Don't hesitate to change providers who don't understand neurodivergence or dismiss your concerns. You deserve knowledgeable, respectful care. Ask potential providers about their experience with autism and ADHD in women during initial consultations.

Coordinating Care

Professional support teams work best when members communicate with each other. Sign releases allowing your providers to share relevant information. This prevents contradictory recommendations and ensures everyone understands your complete picture.

Schedule regular check-ins with core team members even when you're doing well. Prevention is easier than crisis management, and maintaining relationships during stable periods makes getting help during difficult times much smoother.

Consider appointing a care coordinator if your needs are complex. This might be your primary care physician, a case manager through insurance, or a family member who helps manage appointments and communication between providers.

Sustaining Your Network Over Time

Network Maintenance

Support networks require ongoing attention to remain healthy and functional. People's needs change, life circumstances shift, and group dynamics evolve. Regular assessment helps you recognize when adjustments are needed.

Schedule periodic reviews of your support system. Who provides emotional support versus practical help? Where are the gaps? Which relationships energize you versus drain you? This information guides decisions about where to invest your limited social energy.

Maintain reciprocity in your relationships when possible. You don't need to match exactly what others provide, but contributing your strengths helps relationships feel balanced. Maybe you're excellent at research and can share resources, or you have professional skills others need.

Managing Burnout and Boundaries

Social support can become overwhelming, especially for AuDHD women who struggle with people-pleasing or have difficulty recognizing their limits. Set clear boundaries about availability, communication methods, and the type of support you can provide others.

Create systems that prevent overcommitment. Use calendars to schedule social recovery time, set limits on daily messages or calls, and practice saying no to requests that exceed your capacity.

Recognize signs that your support network is becoming a source of stress rather than help. These might include dreading group meetings, feeling obligated to solve everyone's problems, or experiencing increased anxiety around network members.

Building Bridges Between Different Support Systems

Your various support systems - online communities, local groups, family, and professionals - can sometimes feel disconnected or even contradictory. Learning to integrate these different sources of support maximizes their effectiveness while minimizing conflicts.

Share relevant insights between systems when appropriate. Information from your online community might help your therapist understand your experience better. Strategies from your support group could benefit family members. Professional recommendations might be valuable to share in peer communities.

However, maintain appropriate boundaries. Don't share personal details from therapy in peer groups, or expect family members to provide the same type of support as trained professionals. Each system serves different purposes in your overall support network.

Key Insights for Network Building

Your support network is not a luxury - it's a necessity for thriving as an AuDHD woman. Here are the essential takeaways from building this foundation:

- **Start online but don't stop there** - Digital communities provide immediate connection and understanding, but local relationships offer practical support and face-to-face interaction
- **Quality trumps quantity** - A few deep, understanding relationships serve you better than many superficial connections
- **Education is ongoing** - Teaching others about your needs is not a one-time conversation but an ongoing process that requires patience and persistence
- **Professional support is specialized** - Seek providers with specific training in autism and ADHD in women, not just general mental health or medical knowledge
- **Boundaries protect your energy** - Clear limits on your availability and the support you provide others prevent burnout and maintain healthy relationships
- **Integration maximizes effectiveness** - Your various support systems work best when they complement rather than compete with each other

Building your support network takes time, energy, and courage. You'll encounter setbacks, disappointing relationships, and moments when you question if the effort is worth it. But the women who persist in creating these connections find that their support network becomes the foundation for every other positive change in their lives. Your people are out there, waiting to understand and celebrate exactly who you are.

Chapter 12: Embracing Your Authentic Self

The mask you've worn for so long feels heavy now. Years of mimicking others, suppressing your natural responses, and contorting yourself to fit neurotypical expectations have left you exhausted and disconnected from your true self. The journey toward authenticity as an AuDHD woman isn't just about removing this mask - it's about remembering who you were before you learned to hide, and discovering who you can become when you stop apologizing for your neurodivergent brain.

Authenticity for AuDHD women carries unique challenges. Your genuine self might include traits that society has labeled as "too much," "weird," or "inappropriate." Your authentic responses might not match social expectations. Your true needs might inconvenience others. But suppressing these aspects of yourself comes at a cost that becomes too high to bear. The energy spent maintaining false personas could be redirected toward pursuits that actually matter to you.

This chapter isn't about becoming someone new - it's about uncovering who you've always been beneath the layers of masking and accommodation. It's about designing a life that works with your brain instead of against it, and celebrating the strengths that make you uniquely valuable.

Unmasking at Sustainable Paces

Understanding Your Masking Patterns

Before you can unmask effectively, you need to understand how and when you mask. Masking for AuDHD women often begins so early that it feels automatic. You might not realize you're doing it until you're completely drained from the effort.

Common masking behaviors include suppressing stimming, forcing eye contact during conversations, scripting social interactions, mimicking others' interests, hiding sensory sensitivities, and performing neurotypical social behaviors that feel unnatural. You might mask your ADHD by sitting still when you need to move, or mask your autism by engaging in small talk that overwhelms your processing capacity.

Keep a masking journal for two weeks. Note when you feel most authentic versus when you feel like you're performing. Pay attention to the physical sensations of masking - tension in your body, mental fatigue, or emotional numbness. Track which environments, people, and activities trigger your masking behaviors.

Lisa, a 39-year-old librarian, discovered through journaling that she masked most heavily during staff meetings and parent conferences. "I would script responses beforehand, force myself to make eye contact, and suppress my tendency to fidget with my pen. By the end of these interactions, I felt completely drained and needed hours to recover. I hadn't realized how much energy I was spending trying to appear 'normal.'"

Gradual Unmasking Strategies

Unmasking isn't an all-or-nothing process. Dropping all masking behaviors simultaneously can feel overwhelming and may create more problems than it solves. Instead, approach unmasking as a gradual process of authentic self-expression.

Start with low-stakes environments where the consequences of authentic behavior are minimal. This might be at home with understanding family members, in your car during commutes, or in online communities where you feel safe. Practice allowing your natural responses in these spaces before expanding to more challenging environments.

Choose one masking behavior to address at a time. If you typically suppress stimming, begin by allowing small movements like pen-clicking or leg-bouncing in private settings. Once this feels natural, gradually introduce these behaviors in safe social contexts.

Develop scripts for explaining your authentic behaviors to others. "I think better when I move" or "I process information more effectively with written summaries" gives others context for your needs without requiring detailed explanations of your neurodivergence.

Managing Unmasking Anxiety

The prospect of showing your authentic self can trigger intense anxiety. You might worry about rejection, judgment, or negative consequences. These fears are often based on real past experiences of being criticized or excluded for neurodivergent traits.

Practice self-compassion during the unmasking process. Your masking behaviors developed as protective mechanisms, and they served important purposes. You don't need to judge yourself for having masked or for feeling anxious about authentic expression.

Create safety plans for unmasking attempts. Identify supportive people you can contact if you experience negative reactions. Prepare self-care activities for after challenging unmasking experiences. Having these supports in place reduces anxiety about taking authentic risks.

Remember that some people's negative reactions say more about them than about you. Not everyone will understand or appreciate your authentic self, and that's information about their limitations rather than your worth.

Workplace Unmasking Considerations

Workplace unmasking requires particular care because employment consequences can significantly impact your life. Begin by assessing your workplace culture, legal protections, and the openness of your immediate supervisor to neurodiversity discussions.

Start with accommodations that improve your performance rather than just comfort. If you work better with written instructions, request project details via email. If you're more productive with consistent schedules, advocate for predictable meeting times. Frame these requests in terms of work quality rather than personal needs.

Consider partial unmasking in professional settings. You might allow yourself to stim with discrete fidget tools, wear noise-canceling headphones during focused work, or communicate your need for processing time before responding to complex questions.

Document your accommodation requests and any resistance you encounter. If you choose to disclose your neurodivergence formally, having records of your performance and accommodation needs supports your case.

Tamara, a 31-year-old marketing coordinator, began workplace unmasking by requesting written project briefs instead of verbal instructions. When her supervisor saw her project quality improve, she became more open to other accommodations. "I gradually introduced other authentic work styles - standing during long meetings, using a stress ball during conference calls, and scheduling thinking time between back-to-back meetings. Each successful accommodation made the next request easier."

Celebrating Neurodivergent Strengths

Reframing Your Traits

Society often pathologizes neurodivergent traits, focusing on deficits rather than differences. This deficit-focused perspective can make it difficult to recognize and celebrate your strengths. Reframing your traits involves seeing them as neutral differences that can be advantageous in the right contexts.

Hyperfocus, often described as an ADHD "symptom," becomes laser-like concentration that allows you to achieve exceptional results in areas of interest. Attention to detail, sometimes labeled as autistic "rigidity," becomes quality control that catches errors others miss. Sensory sensitivity, frequently seen as a limitation, becomes awareness that allows you to notice subtleties others overlook.

Your tendency to think differently isn't a flaw - it's innovation potential. Your need for routine isn't inflexibility - it's system optimization that frees mental energy for important tasks. Your emotional intensity isn't instability - it's depth that allows for profound connections and experiences.

Create a strengths inventory by listing your natural abilities, interests, and ways of thinking. Include traits that others might see as challenges but that you can recognize as potential advantages. Ask trusted friends and family members to contribute to this list - sometimes others see our strengths more clearly than we do.

Leveraging Strengths in Daily Life

Once you recognize your strengths, the next step is actively incorporating them into your daily routines and major life decisions. This might mean restructuring your schedule to accommodate your natural energy rhythms, choosing career paths that utilize your hyperfocus abilities, or designing your living space to support your sensory needs.

If you have strong pattern recognition skills, use them for problem-solving in your work or personal life. If you excel at systems thinking, apply this to organizing your home or streamlining processes for your family. If you have exceptional memory for specific topics, become the go-to resource in those areas.

Don't apologize for using your strengths, even if they seem unconventional. If you work better with background music, don't justify this need to others. If you prefer written communication for complex topics, present this as a strength rather than a limitation.

Building on Special Interests

Special interests are one of the most misunderstood aspects of autism, often dismissed as obsessions or seen as limiting. In reality, special interests can become gateways to expertise, career success, and deep personal satisfaction.

Your intense interest in specific topics gives you knowledge depth that few people achieve. This expertise can translate into career opportunities, creative projects, or ways to help others. Many successful careers have been built on what started as childhood special interests.

Don't limit yourself to traditional applications of your interests. If you're fascinated by organization systems, you might become a professional organizer, write productivity blogs, or help friends streamline their homes. If you love collecting information about specific topics, you might become a researcher, consultant, or educator in those areas.

Connect your special interests to social opportunities. Join clubs, attend conferences, or participate in online communities related to your interests. These environments often attract other neurodivergent individuals and provide natural conversation topics.

Maya, a 36-year-old graphic designer, turned her childhood special interest in typography into a successful freelance career specializing in accessible design. "What my teachers called 'obsessing over fonts' became expertise that clients pay premium rates for. I can spot readability issues that other designers miss, and I know which typefaces work best for different audiences. My 'obsession' is actually my competitive advantage."

Designing Life Around Your Needs

Environmental Design

Your physical environment significantly impacts your ability to function authentically. Designing spaces that support your sensory needs, organizational style, and work preferences removes barriers to authentic self-expression.

Start with sensory considerations. If fluorescent lights cause discomfort, invest in alternative lighting options. If background noise disrupts your concentration, create quiet zones in your home. If clutter overwhelms your visual processing, develop organizational systems that maintain clear surfaces.

Consider your work style when arranging spaces. If you think better while moving, create areas where pacing or fidgeting is comfortable. If you need visual reminders, design systems that keep important information visible. If you work better with specific materials or tools, organize them for easy access.

Don't apologize for your environmental needs or try to make your spaces look like neurotypical environments. Your home should support your functioning, not impress visitors who don't understand your needs.

Schedule Design

Traditional schedules often conflict with AuDHD energy patterns and processing needs. Designing your schedule around your natural rhythms improves both productivity and well-being.

Identify your optimal times for different types of activities. Many AuDHD women have specific periods when they're most creative, most social, or most able to handle administrative tasks. Schedule important activities during these peak periods when possible.

Build in transition time between activities, especially those requiring different types of processing. If you're switching from a social interaction to focused work, allow time to decompress and shift mental gears.

Include regular time for special interests, sensory regulation, and processing. These aren't luxuries - they're maintenance activities that keep your system functioning optimally.

Relationship Design

Authentic relationships require people who accept and appreciate your neurodivergent traits. This doesn't mean surrounding yourself only with other neurodivergent people, but it does mean choosing relationships with individuals who respect your differences.

Communicate your needs clearly in relationships. Explain how you process emotions, what types of support help you most, and what overwhelms you. Give others specific information about how to interact with you successfully.

Set boundaries that protect your energy and authentic self-expression. This might mean limiting social commitments during overwhelming periods, asking for written communication about complex topics, or requesting advance notice for social plans.

Don't try to change fundamental aspects of yourself to maintain relationships. If someone requires you to mask constantly or dismiss your needs, the relationship isn't sustainable or healthy.

Letters to Younger Selves

Healing Through Self-Compassion

Writing letters to your younger self can be a powerful healing exercise that addresses the internalized shame and confusion many AuDHD women carry from childhood experiences of being different.

Your letter might address the child who was told to sit still when her body needed to move, the teenager who felt like an alien among her peers, or the young adult who struggled with life transitions that seemed easy for others. Offer the understanding and validation that younger version of yourself needed but didn't receive.

Explain what you know now about neurodivergence that would have helped then. Describe how her differences aren't flaws but variations that will become strengths. Reassure her that the struggle to fit in isn't her fault and that she will eventually find her people.

Sarah's letter to her teenage self included this passage: "That intensity you feel about your interests isn't something to hide - it's your superpower. The other kids might not understand why you care so much about marine biology, but that passion will carry you through college, graduate school, and into a career you love. Stop trying to tone yourself down to fit in. The right people will appreciate your enthusiasm."

Acknowledging Growth and Resilience

Your letter can also acknowledge the incredible resilience and adaptation you've demonstrated throughout your life. Recognize the strength it took to navigate a world designed for neurotypical brains, often without understanding why things felt so difficult.

Celebrate the coping strategies you developed, even if they weren't perfect. Your masking behaviors served important protective functions. Your people-pleasing tendencies showed your desire to connect with others. Your perfectionism reflected your high standards and attention to quality.

Acknowledge the pain you experienced without minimizing it. Feeling different, misunderstood, or excluded creates real trauma that deserves recognition and healing. Validating these experiences helps you process them and move forward.

Sharing Wisdom and Hope

Include in your letter the wisdom you've gained about living authentically as an AuDHD woman. Share the strategies that work, the people who understand, and the environments where you thrive. Offer hope that life becomes more manageable as self-understanding increases.

Describe the joy that comes with authentic self-expression - the relief of stimming when you need to, the satisfaction of pursuing your interests deeply, the peace of being around people who accept you completely. These positive experiences can motivate continued growth and self-acceptance.

End your letter with specific encouragement and love. Many AuDHD women struggle with self-criticism and perfectionism. Offering yourself the unconditional love and acceptance you needed can be transformative.

Making the Abstract Concrete

Consider making your letter actionable by including specific advice your younger self could have used. What accommodations would have helped in school? Which relationships should have been prioritized or avoided? What self-care practices would have made difficult periods more manageable?

This practical guidance helps you consolidate your learning and creates a resource you can reference during current challenges. Sometimes the advice you would give your younger self applies directly to present situations.

Create a ritual around your letter-writing. Choose a meaningful location, set aside uninterrupted time, and treat the process with the reverence it deserves. Consider sharing portions of your letter with trusted friends or family members who might benefit from understanding your experience better.

Jessica, a 44-year-old social worker, wrote multiple letters to herself at different ages. "Writing to my eight-year-old self helped me understand why I developed such strong people-pleasing tendencies. The letter to my college-age self addressed the shame I felt about struggling with things that seemed easy for others. Each letter helped me process a different layer of my experience and offer myself the compassion I needed."

Living Your Values Authentically

Identifying Core Values

Authentic living requires clarity about your core values - the principles that guide your decisions and define what matters most to you. For many AuDHD women, years of masking and people-pleasing can obscure these values, making it difficult to distinguish between what you truly believe and what you think you should believe.

Reflect on moments when you felt most authentic and fulfilled. What values were you honoring in those situations? Consider times when you felt particularly distressed or conflicted - often these feelings indicate value conflicts or situations where you're not living according to your principles.

Common values for many AuDHD women include authenticity, justice, deep connections, learning, creativity, and helping others. Your specific combination of values is unique and might not match typical societal priorities. This is normal and healthy.

Aligning Actions with Values

Once you identify your core values, assess how well your current life aligns with them. Are you spending time and energy on activities that reflect what matters most to you? Are your relationships, work, and daily routines consistent with your values?

Identify areas where your actions don't match your values and develop plans for better alignment. This might involve career changes, relationship adjustments, or shifts in how you spend your free time. Small changes can have significant impacts on overall life satisfaction.

Don't expect perfect alignment immediately. Living authentically is an ongoing process of adjustment and growth. Focus on gradual improvements rather than dramatic overhauls.

Embracing Your Journey Forward

Living authentically as an AuDHD woman is not a destination but an ongoing process of discovery, acceptance, and growth. You will have setbacks, moments of doubt, and times when masking feels necessary for survival. This doesn't mean you're failing - it means you're human.

Your authentic self is not fixed or unchanging. As you grow and learn, your understanding of yourself will evolve. The person you are today might be different from who you were when you first learned about your neurodivergence, and that's perfectly normal.

Trust the process of becoming yourself. The world needs your unique perspective, your deep thinking, your passionate interests, and your genuine way of being. By living authentically, you give other AuDHD women permission to do the same.

Essential Points for Authentic Living

Your journey toward authentic self-expression as an AuDHD woman requires patience, courage, and self-compassion. Here are the crucial insights for embracing your true self:

- **Unmask gradually and strategically** - Start in safe environments and expand slowly, always prioritizing your safety and well-being
- **Reframe traits as differences, not deficits** - Your neurodivergent characteristics are variations that can become advantages in the right contexts
- **Design your environment to support authenticity** - Create spaces, schedules, and relationships that work with your brain rather than against it
- **Use special interests as strengths** - Your intense interests can become expertise, career opportunities, and sources of deep satisfaction
- **Honor your core values** - Authentic living requires knowing what matters most to you and aligning your actions accordingly
- **Practice self-compassion** - Healing the wounds of feeling different requires treating yourself with the kindness you deserved all along

The mask you've worn served important purposes, protecting you when you didn't have other options. But now you have knowledge, strategies, and hopefully a support network that makes authentic living possible. Your genuine self - with all your quirks, intensities, and beautiful differences - deserves to exist freely in this world. The journey toward authenticity isn't always easy, but it's the path to a life that truly belongs to you.

References

1. Attwood, T., & Gray, C. (2019). The Complete Guide to Asperger's Syndrome: Revised Edition. Jessica Kingsley Publishers.
2. Gaines, K., Bourne, L., Pearson, M., & Kleijer, M. (2016). "Women with autism spectrum conditions: Exploring the impact of masking." Autism Research, 9(6), 732-744.
3. Hull, L., Petrides, K. V., Allison, C., Smith, P., Baron-Cohen, S., Lai, M. C., & Mandy, W. (2017). "Putting on my best normal": Social camouflaging in adults with autism spectrum conditions. Journal of Autism and Developmental Disorders, 47(8), 2519-2534.
4. Lai, M. C., Lombardo, M. V., Ruigrok, A. N., Chakrabarti, B., Auyeung, B., Szatmari, P., ... & Baron-Cohen, S. (2017). Quantifying and exploring camouflaging in men and women with autism. Autism, 21(6), 690-702.
5. Loomes, R., Hull, L., & Mandy, W. P. L. (2017). What is the male-to-female ratio in autism spectrum disorder? A systematic review and meta-analysis. Journal of the American Academy of Child & Adolescent Psychiatry, 56(6), 466-474.
6. Mowery, D. L., Dedrick, R. F., & Epstein, M. H. (2015). The relationship between ADHD and autism spectrum disorders: A systematic review. Research in Autism Spectrum Disorders, 12, 82-91.
7. Quinn, P. O., & Madhavan, S. (2014). A review of attention-deficit/hyperactivity disorder in women and girls: Uncovering this hidden diagnosis. The Primary Care Companion for CNS Disorders, 16(3).
8. Rynkiewicz, A., Schuller, B., Marchi, E., Piana, S., Camurri, A., Lassalle, A., & Baron-Cohen, S. (2016). An investigation of the 'female camouflaging effect' in autism using a computerized ADOS-2 and a test of sex/gender differences. Molecular Autism, 7(1), 10.
9. Sedgewick, F., Hill, V., Yates, R., Pickering, L., & Pellicano, E. (2016). Gender differences in the social motivation and friendship experiences of autistic and non-autistic adolescents.

Journal of Autism and Developmental Disorders, 46(4), 1297-1306.

10. Young, S., Bramham, J., Gray, K., & Rose, E. (2018). The experience of receiving a diagnosis and treatment of ADHD in adulthood: A qualitative study of clinically referred patients using interpretative phenomenological analysis. Journal of Attention Disorders, 22(11), 1071-1084.

11. ADHD After Pregnancy: What to Expect. (2023). Healthline. Retrieved from https://www.healthline.com/health/pregnancy/adhd-after-pregnancy

12. ADHD and Hormones: ADD Symptoms in Teen Girls, Women. (2025). ADDitude Magazine. Retrieved from https://www.additudemag.com/women-hormones-and-adhd/

13. ADHD and Hormones in Women. Relational Psych. Retrieved from https://www.relationalpsych.group/articles/adhd-and-hormones-in-women

14. ADHD and Menopause: Changing Symptoms and Treatments. (2022). Healthline. Retrieved from https://www.healthline.com/health/menopause/adhd-and-menopause

15. ADHD and perinatal mental health: Breaking the silence for neurodivergent mothers. Maternal Mental Health Alliance. Retrieved from https://maternalmentalhealthalliance.org/news/adhd-perinatal-mental-health-breaking-silence-neurodivergent-mothers/

16. ADHD in Adults: 4 Things to Know. National Institute of Mental Health (NIMH). Retrieved from https://www.nimh.nih.gov/health/publications/adhd-what-you-need-to-know

17. ADHD Masking: Does Hiding Your Symptoms Help or Harm? - ADDA - Attention Deficit Disorder Association. (2025). Retrieved from https://add.org/adhd-masking/

18. ADHD, Autism, and Women in Menopause. Bristol Menopause. Retrieved from https://www.bristolmenopause.com/news/adhd,-autism,-and-women-in-menopause

19. Adults With Executive Function Disorder. (2024). The OT Toolbox. Retrieved from https://www.theottoolbox.com/adults-executive-function-disorder/

20. As An Autistic Mum, Pregnancy And Motherhood Is A Sensory Overload. (2024). HuffPost UK Parents. Retrieved from https://www.huffingtonpost.co.uk/entry/as-an-autistic-mum-pregnancy-and-motherhood-is-a-sensory-overload_uk_65c351e4e4b0dbc806aeb66f

21. Associations Between ADHD Symptoms and Maternal and Birth Outcomes. PMC. Retrieved from https://pmc.ncbi.nlm.nih.gov/articles/PMC9597155/

22. Attention-deficit/hyperactivity disorder and the menstrual cycle: Theory and evidence. (2023). ScienceDirect. Retrieved from https://www.sciencedirect.com/science/article/abs/pii/S0018506X23001642

23. Attention Deficit Hyperactivity Disorder (ADHD) and the menopause transition. (2024). My Menopause Centre. Retrieved from https://www.mymenopausecentre.com/gp-resources/attention-deficit-hyperactivity-disorder-adhd-and-the-menopause-transition/

24. Attention-Deficit/Hyperactivity Disorder: What You Need to Know. National Institute of Mental Health (NIMH). Retrieved from https://www.nimh.nih.gov/health/publications/attention-deficit-hyperactivity-disorder-what-you-need-to-know

25. AuDHD - Autistic Girls Network. (2024). Retrieved from https://autisticgirlsnetwork.org/audhd/

26. AuDHD in Women: From Masking to Mastery. Udemy. Retrieved from https://www.udemy.com/course/audhd-in-women-from-masking-to-mastery/

27. AuDHD, sensory meltdowns, and hormones (Sam Hiew's story). (2024). Understood. Retrieved from https://www.understood.org/en/podcasts/adhd-aha/audhd-sensory-meltdowns-samantha-hiew

28. Autism and Pregnancy: Navigating Motherhood on the Spectrum. (2024). NeuroLaunch. Retrieved from https://neurolaunch.com/autism-and-pregnancy/

29. Autism and puberty aggression. Autism Speaks. Retrieved from https://www.autismspeaks.org/expert-opinion/autism-puberty-aggression

30. Autism, Adolescence and Hormones. Attwood & Garnett Events. Retrieved from https://www.attwoodandgarnettevents.com/blogs/news/autism-adolescence-and-hormones

31. Being a Woman Is 100% Significant to My Experiences of Attention Deficit Hyperactivity Disorder and Autism. (2024). PubMed. Retrieved from https://pubmed.ncbi.nlm.nih.gov/39025117/

32. Being a Woman Is 100% Significant to My Experiences of Attention Deficit Hyperactivity Disorder and Autism. (2024). Retrieved from https://pmc.ncbi.nlm.nih.gov/articles/PMC11580322/

33. Boys vs. Girls: How Puberty Affects ADHD Symptoms. (2024). ADDitude Magazine. Retrieved from https://www.additudemag.com/puberty-and-adhd-symptoms-teens/

34. Camouflage and masking behavior in adult autism. (2023). Frontiers in Psychiatry. Retrieved from https://www.frontiersin.org/journals/psychiatry/articles/10.3389/fpsyt.2023.1108110/full

35. College, career, commitment, oh my: how emerging adult women balance romantic relationships, career plans, and financial stability. Clark University. Retrieved from https://commons.clarku.edu/faculty_psychology/23/

36. Dopamine, Estrogen and ADHD. (2023). Adult ADHD Centre. Retrieved from https://adultadhdcentre.com/article/dopamine-estrogen-and-adhd/

37. Exclusion of females in autism research: Empirical evidence for a "leaky" recruitment-to-research pipeline. PMC. Retrieved from https://pmc.ncbi.nlm.nih.gov/articles/PMC9804357/

38. Executive Function Coaching for Adults. (2023). BrainCog. Retrieved from https://www.braincogcoach.com/executive-function-coaching-for-adults/

39. Finding Work That Works For You: A Career Guide for Young Adults with ADHD. (2023). Executive Function

Specialists. Retrieved from
https://www.efspecialists.com/post/workingwithadhd

40. Hormonal Changes and ADHD: Symptoms Through the Lifespan. (2023). ADDitude Magazine. Retrieved from https://www.additudemag.com/hormonal-changes-adhd-puberty-postpartum-menopause-andropause/

41. How Does Menopause Affect ADHD? (2024). WebMD. Retrieved from https://www.webmd.com/add-adhd/adhd-and-menopause

42. How hormones and the menstrual cycle can affect women with ADHD. (2023). Monash Lens. Retrieved from https://lens.monash.edu/@medicine-health/2023/09/24/1386049/how-hormones-and-the-menstrual-cycle-can-affect-women-with-adhd-5-common-questions

43. How Puberty and ADHD Interact and Compound Symptoms. (2025). ADDitude Magazine. Retrieved from https://www.additudemag.com/puberty-and-adhd/

44. Is it ADHD, Menopause or Autism? (2023). Living on The Spectrum. Retrieved from https://www.livingonthespectrum.com/health-and-wellbeing/autism-adhd-menopause/

45. Masking. Autism.org.uk. Retrieved from https://www.autism.org.uk/advice-and-guidance/topics/behaviour/masking

46. Menopause. Autism.org.uk. Retrieved from https://www.autism.org.uk/advice-and-guidance/topics/physical-health/menopause

47. Menopause, Hormones & ADHD: What We Know, What Research is Needed. (2022). ADDitude Magazine. Retrieved from https://www.additudemag.com/menopause-hormones-adhd-women-research/

48. Menopause Symptoms Exacerbate ADHD in Women: ADDitude Survey. (2022). ADDitude Magazine. Retrieved from https://www.additudemag.com/menopause-symptoms-adhd-survey/

49. Miss. Diagnosis: A Systematic Review of ADHD in Adult Women. PMC. Retrieved from https://pmc.ncbi.nlm.nih.gov/articles/PMC10173330/

50. Parental ADHD in pregnancy and the postpartum period - A systematic review. PubMed. Retrieved from https://pubmed.ncbi.nlm.nih.gov/33516734/
51. Parenting as a New Autistic Mother: The Impact on Daily Living. Neurodivergent Insights. Retrieved from https://neurodivergentinsights.com/autistic-mothers/
52. Perimenopause Problems: How Changing Hormones Exacerbate ADHD Symptoms. (2023). ADDitude Magazine. Retrieved from https://www.additudemag.com/add-and-menopause-how-hormones-affect-adhd-symptoms/
53. Postpartum Care for Mothers with ADHD: A Guide for Clinicians. (2024). ADDitude Magazine. Retrieved from https://www.additudemag.com/postpartum-care-adhd-clinician-guide/
54. The 16 Best Jobs for Creative & Restless ADHD Brains. (2016). ADDitude Magazine. Retrieved from https://www.additudemag.com/slideshows/jobs-for-people-with-adhd/
55. The Autistic Doula: Navigating the Sensory Challenges of Motherhood. (2023). Reframing Autism. Retrieved from https://reframingautism.org.au/the-autistic-doula-navigating-the-sensory-challenges-of-motherhood/
56. The Best Jobs for People with ADHD. (2022). Psych Central. Retrieved from https://psychcentral.com/adhd/best-jobs-for-people-with-adhd
57. The Best Jobs for People with ADHD. (2024). WebMD. Retrieved from https://www.webmd.com/add-adhd/best-jobs-adults
58. The Complete Picture: How Estrogen Affects Women with ADHD. (2018). CHADD. Retrieved from https://chadd.org/adhd-weekly/the-complete-picture-how-estrogen-affects-women-with-adhd/
59. The Cost of Camouflage: Understanding Masking in ADHD, Autistic, and AuDHD Adults. (2025). Myndset Therapeutics. Retrieved from https://www.myndset-therapeutics.com/post/the-cost-of-camouflage
60. The Different Signs Of AuDHD In Women & Girls. Augmentive. Retrieved from https://augmentive.io/blog/signs-audhd-women-girls

61. The Role of Estrogen Receptors and Their Signaling across Psychiatric Disorders. (2020). MDPI. Retrieved from https://www.mdpi.com/1422-0067/22/1/373

62. Those Lovely 'Mones: The Intersection of ADHD and Hormones. (2023). CHADD. Retrieved from https://chadd.org/adhd-news/adhd-news-adults/attention-those-lovely-mones-the-intersection-of-adhd-and-hormones/

63. Understanding Autism and ADHD in Women. (2025). Autism Parenting Magazine. Retrieved from https://www.autismparentingmagazine.com/autism-and-adhd-in-women/

64. Understanding Autism Masking and Its Consequences. (2021). Healthline. Retrieved from https://www.healthline.com/health/autism/autism-masking

65. Understanding the Unique Challenges of Autistic Mothers. (2024). Psychology Today. Retrieved from https://www.psychologytoday.com/us/blog/the-neurodivergent-psychologist/202405/understanding-the-unique-challenges-of-autistic-mothers

66. Unmasking Autism and ADHD in Women. Sachs Center. Retrieved from https://sachscenter.com/autism-and-adhd-in-women/

67. What is Executive Function Coaching. Beyond BookSmart. Retrieved from https://www.beyondbooksmart.com/what-is-ef-coaching

68. What is puberty like for teens with ADHD? ADHD and teenagers. Retrieved from https://parents.au.reachout.com/mental-health-and-wellbeing/adhd/what-is-puberty-like-for-teens-with-adhd

69. Women and ADHD: How menopause can affect women with ADHD. (2023). Psych-UK Limited. Retrieved from https://psychiatry-uk.com/women-and-adhd-how-menopause-can-affect-women-with-adhd/

70. Women in Autism. (2024). Autism Research Institute. Retrieved from https://autism.org/women-in-autism/

71. Women with autism & ADHD aren't diagnosed until adulthood. (2022). Durham University. Retrieved from https://www.durham.ac.uk/research/current/thought-

leadership/women-with-autism--adhd-arent-diagnosed-until-adulthood/

72. Women's higher health risks in the obesogenic environment: a gender nutrition approach to metabolic dimorphism with predictive, preventive, and personalised medicine. PMC. Retrieved from https://pmc.ncbi.nlm.nih.gov/articles/PMC3560240/

www.ingramcontent.com/pod-product-compliance
Lightning Source LLC
Chambersburg PA
CBHW071225290326
41931CB00037B/1974